FIRST PLACE BIBLE

D0366214

Healthy BOUNDARIES

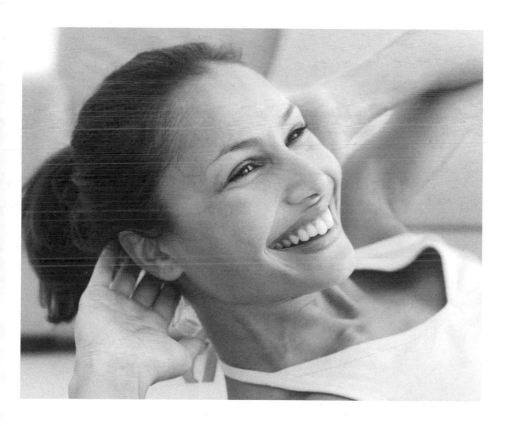

Gospel Light

FIRST PLACE™

Gospel Light is a Christian publisher dedicated to serving the local church. We believe God's vision for Gospel Light is to provide church leaders with biblical, user-friendly materials that will help them evangelize, disciple and minister to children, youth and families.

It is our prayer that this Gospel Light resource will help you discover biblical truth for your own life and help you minister to others. May God richly bless you.

For a free catalog of resources from Gospel Light, please contact your Christian supplier or contact us at 1-800-4-GOSPEL or www.gospellight.com.

PUBLISHING STAFF
William T. Greig, Publisher • **Dr. Elmer L. Towns,** Senior Consulting Publisher • **Bayard Taylor, M.Div.,** Senior Editor, Biblical and Theological Issues • **Elizabeth Crews,** Contributing Writer

---

CAUTION
The information contained in this book is intended to be solely informational and educational. It is assumed that the First Place participant will consult a medical or health professional before beginning this or any other weight-loss or physical fitness program.

CONTENTS

FOREWORD

My introduction to Bible study came when I joined First Place in March 1981. I had been in church since I was a small child, but the extent of my study of the Bible had been reading my Sunday School quarterly on Saturday night. On Sunday morning, I would listen to my Sunday School teacher as she taught God's Word to me. During the worship service, I would listen to our pastor as he taught God's Word to me. Digging out the truths of the Bible for myself had frankly never entered my mind.

Perhaps you are right where I was back in 1981. If so, you are in for a blessing you never dreamed possible. As you start studying the truths of the Bible for yourself, you will see God begin to open your understanding of His Word. Bible study is one of the Nine Commitments of the First Place program. The First Place Bible studies are designed to be done on a daily basis. Each day's study will take approximately 15 to 20 minutes to complete, but you will be discovering the deep truths of God's Word as you work through each week's study.

There are many in-depth Bible studies on the market. The First Place Bible studies are not designed for the purpose of in-depth study. They are designed to be used in conjunction with the other eight commitments of the program to bring balance into our lives. Our desire is for each member to begin having a personal quiet time with God each day. This time alone with God should include a time of prayer, Bible reading and Bible study. Having a quiet time is a daily discipline that will bring the rich rewards of balance, something we all need.

A part of each week's study is the Bible memory verse for the week. Almost every First Place member I have talked with about the program says, "The weight loss is wonderful, but the most important thing I have received from my association with First Place is learning to study God's Word."

God bless you as you begin this exciting journey toward a balanced life. God will richly bless your efforts to give Him first place in your life. Remember Matthew 6:33: "But seek first his kingdom and his righteousness, and all these things will be given to you as well."

Carole Lewis
First Place National Director

INTRODUCTION

The First Place Bible studies were developed to be used in conjunction with the First Place weight-loss program. However, the studies could also be used by anyone who desires to learn more about God's Word and His will, with the added bonus of learning more about living a healthy lifestyle.

A Balanced Life

First Place is a Christ-centered health program, emphasizing balance in the physical, mental, emotional and spiritual areas of life. The First Place program is meant to be a daily process. As we learn to keep Christ first in our lives, we will find that He is the One who satisfies our hunger and our every need.

God's Word contains guidelines for maintaining our physical well-being, equipping us mentally to make right choices, providing emotional stability to handle everyday circumstances as well as crisis situations and growing spiritually as we deepen our relationship with Him.

The Nine Commitments

The First Place program has Nine Commitments that will help you draw closer to the Lord and aid you in establishing a solid, consistent and healthy Christian life. Each commitment is a necessary and important part of the goal of First Place to help you become healthier and stronger in all areas of your life—living the abundant life He has planned for each of us. To help you achieve growth in all four areas, First Place asks you to keep these Nine Commitments:

1. Attendance
2. Encouragement
3. Prayer
4. Bible Reading
5. Scripture Memory Verse
6. Bible study
7. Live-It Plan
8. Commitment Record
9. Exercise

The Components

There are 5 distinct components to this Bible study to aid you in bringing balance to your life. These components include the 10-week Bible study, 4 Wellness Worksheets, 2 weeks of menu plans, the leader's discussion guide and 13 Commitment Records.

The Bible Study

Each week of each 10-week Bible study is divided into five daily assignments with Days 6 and 7 set aside for reflections on the week's lesson. The following guidelines will help make your study more enjoyable and profitable:

- Set aside 15 to 20 minutes each day to complete the daily assignment. It's best not to attempt to complete a week's worth of Bible study in one day.
- Pray before each day's study and ask God to give you understanding and a teachable heart.
- Keep in mind that the ultimate goal of Bible study is not only for knowledge but also for application and a changed life.
- First Place suggests using the *New International Version* of the Bible to complete the studies.
- Don't feel anxious if you can't seem to find the *correct* answer. Many times the Word will speak differently to different people, depending upon where they are in their walk with God and the season of life they are experiencing.
- Be prepared to discuss with your fellow First Place members what you learned that week through your study.

Wellness Worksheets

This study's Wellness Worksheets are interactive and will help you further explore the topic of becoming a new creation in Christ.

Menu Plans

The two-week menu plans were developed especially for First Place by Chef Scott Wilson. Each menu is meant to simplify meal planning and include food exchanges. These meals are based on the MasterCook software that uses a database of over 6,000 food items and was prepared using United States Department of Agriculture (USDA) publications and information from food manufacturers.

Leader's Discussion Guide

This discussion guide is provided to help the First Place leader guide a group through this Bible study. It provides information for the leader to prepare for each weekly group meeting.

Personal Weight Record

The Personal Weight Record is for the member to use to keep a record of weight loss. After the weigh-in at each week's meeting, the member will record any loss or gain on the chart.

Commitment Records

Thirteen Commitment Records (CRs) are provided in the back of this Bible study. For your convenience these have been printed on perforated paper so that you can easily remove them from the book and carry them with you through each week as you keep your First Place commitments. Directions for filling out the CRs precede those pages.

ACKNOWLEDGE
THE TRUTH

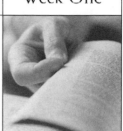

MEMORY VERSE
Then you will know the truth,
and the truth will set you free
John 8:32

All positive change begins by first acknowledging the truth. Jesus Christ
is the way, the truth and the life (see John 14:6). He came so that we can
know the truth and be restored to a right relationship with God. By knowing the truth, we can then cooperate with God as He works to repair our
broken lives, restore our integrity and bestow on us our heritage as His
dearly beloved children. Since the beginning, Satan, the father of lies,
has used his deceptive wiles to keep us enslaved. This week we will look
at the importance of being honest with ourselves and embracing the truth.
We will also examine several pitfalls that keep us from acknowledging the
truth that can set us free: distortion, denial, delusion and disguise.

DAY 1: *What Is Truth?*

Just before handing Jesus over to be crucified, Pilot asked the question
that has echoed throughout salvation history: "What is truth?" (John 18:38).
In today's hi-tech, information-crazed society, we often have trouble distinguishing between truth and falsity. Many different voices compete for
our attention and affirmation, yet for those of us who are in Christ Jesus,
there need be no confusion about truth. Jesus tells His followers that if we
hold to His teaching, we will know the truth and the truth will set us free.

➤ In the prologue to John's Gospel, the beloved disciple introduces us to Jesus, the Word made flesh. Read John 1:1-18 and summarize what John tells us about Jesus Christ in verse 14.

➤ Look up Matthew 11:11, Mark 3:28, Luke 18:17 and John 5:24. What common phrase did Jesus use in all four statements?

While He was here on Earth, Jesus always told His listeners the truth, even in the face of opposition. As He was preparing to go back to His Father in heaven, Jesus told His disciples about another truth teller.

➤ What do the following verses tell us about the one Jesus promised to send in His stead?

John 14:16-17

John 15:26

John 16:13

The Holy Spirit will guide us into all truth if we will listen to His still, small voice amid the noise and confusion of the world. During your quiet time today, listen for His voice. Record in the following space the truth He reveals to you regarding your participation in the First Place program:

➤ What can you do to turn that truth into action?

Father, thank You for sending Jesus, the Word made flesh, into this world so that I can know the truth that will set me free.

Lord, I acknowledge the Holy Spirit as my counselor and guide as I begin to put Your truth into practice in my life.

DAY 2: The Enemy of Truth, Part 1

Jesus warned His followers about the dangers of not hearing and not acknowledging His truth. We face an enemy who is intent on leading the whole world astray.

➤ Read John 8:42-47. Who are the two fathers described in these verses?

➤ In your own words, why does the devil lie (v. 44)?

➤ In stark contrast to the deceitful words spoken by the devil and his children, what do you think characterizes the speech of God's children? Confirm your answer by looking up Ephesians 4:15.

Distinguishing God's truth from Satan's lies would be easy if the devil told blatant, bold-faced lies; however, he is much too clever for that. Instead of telling obvious falsehoods, Satan relies on the subtlety of distortion, denial, delusion and disguise to deceive us.

"**Distortion**" means "taking the truth and slightly changing it into a partial truth"—which, by definition, is no longer truth at all. Truth can also be distorted by pulling Scripture verses out of context so that the words do not convey a complete thought, or by using verses of Scripture in a way that contradicts the whole truth of God's Word. Satan used this tactic when he tempted Jesus in the desert. Look up the three verses below to compare Satan's words with the Scripture Jesus quoted.

- **What Satan said**—Matthew 4:5-7
- **The Scripture he distorted**—Psalm 91:11-12
- **The Scripture Jesus quoted**—Deuteronomy 6:16

Not only did the devil omit part of Psalm 91:11-12 ("to guard you in all your ways"), but also he conveniently omitted the truth of Deuteronomy 6:16: We are not to put God to the test by willfully engaging in foolish, risk-taking behavior.

➤ How was Jesus able to rebuke the tempter's lie?

≫ What can we learn from this encounter about the importance of knowing God's whole truth, rather than picking and choosing verses that suit our purposes?

 Gracious God and Father, thank You for teaching me to speak Your native language.

Help me, O my Father, never to distort the truth of Your Word but rather to devote myself to learning the truth that will set me free.

DAY 3: *The Enemy of Truth, Part 2*

In addition to distorting God's Truth, the evil one uses other weapons from his "Deadly D" arsenal of lies to keep God's children from acknowledging the truth.

"**Denial**" is a word we hear often these days. "Denial" means "refusing to accept or believe the truth."

≫ In Romans 1:18-23, the apostle Paul gives a vivid description of denial. What were these foolish men and women denying?

Though our denial is perhaps not as radical as Paul's description, we all have times when we don't glorify God as God, give Him thanks or acknowledge Him as the Lord of our lives.

≫ How does denial affect your participation in the First Place program?

"**Delusion**" means "the belief in something that contradicts an established fact." Genesis 3:1-5 tells the story of Eve's delusion. Read the passage before answering the following questions.

➤ What was the truth (fact) that Eve chose not to believe?

➤ What did Satan use to blind Eve to the truth?

➤ Share a specific time when Satan used your desire to ignore God's truth, and thus be equal with God in knowledge and power, to tempt you into disobeying God's Word.

➤ Read 1 Corinthians 3:16-17. Are there any beliefs you hold about caring for your body that run contrary to the established truth of God's Word?

"**Disguise**" means "camouflaging a lie so that it resembles truth." Satan is a master of disguise. Look up the following Scriptures to see how Satan takes on different appearances. Record your findings.

Scripture	Satan's Disguise
Genesis 3:1	
2 Corinthians 11:14	
1 Peter 5:8	
Revelation 12:9	

Temptation is always an invitation to fill a legitimate, God-given need through illegitimate means. Satan dangles the bait in front of us much like a fisher dangles a plastic lure disguised as a real worm. Hunger is a legitimate need, but a plastic worm cannot satisfy the fish's true need.

➣ What disguise does Satan use to tempt you to fill your legitimate hunger and thirst for God with things that can't satisfy your need to be in a right relationship with Him?

➣ How can the First Place Scripture memory commitment help you know the truth so that you won't fall prey to Satan's "Deadly Ds"?

 Lord God Almighty, Satan's tools of deception are powerful, but Your truth is stronger than any lie he can tell. Help me cling to Your truth so that I will be shielded from the devil's schemes.

Sovereign Lord, I acknowledge You as the One who created all things. I am without excuse when I do not honor You as my Lord and Savior [see Romans 1:20].

DAY 4: *Paradoxical Truth*

A paradox is a statement that appears to contradict itself, but it is really a truth applied to a deeper level of our being. In Scripture, paradoxes may seem confusing when we try to interpret spiritual truth based on physical reality. Early in John's Gospel we are introduced to Nicodemus, who can help us understand the truth about spiritual paradoxes.

➣ After reading John 3:1-4, summarize Nicodemus's confusion.

➣ In response to Nicodemus's question, Jesus tells him a profound spiritual truth (vv. 5-6). If Nicodemus were standing in the room with you right now, how would you explain to him what it means to be born again?

Scripture contains other paradoxical statements. Look up each of the following verses and then write down the truth and the seeming contradiction:

Scripture	If I Want to...	I Must...
Matthew 5:3		
Luke 9:24		
2 Corinthians 12:9-10		
1 Peter 5:6		

➣ Which of these four paradoxes is hardest for you to understand and apply to your life within the First Place program?

Nicodemus brought his confusion to Jesus, believing He was a great teacher, sent from God. Do you believe that Jesus, the living Word of God, can answer all your questions too? Write a prayer acknowledging the truth of God's Word. In that prayer, be honest with Jesus about your struggle to apply His truth to your First Place program commitments.

My Lord and my God, I confess I am slow to come to You when I do not understand Your Word. Help me to sit at Jesus' feet and learn from Him so that I will not be confused by seeming contradictions.

O Sovereign Lord, when I humble myself under Your mighty hand, I can rest assured You will lift me up in Your time and in Your way [see 1 Peter 5:6].

DAY 5: *The Whole Truth*

Once you accept Jesus Christ as your Lord and Savior and invite Him to be the Lord of your life, your life is then characterized by three actions: justification, sanctification and glorification.

Our life in Christ begins with **justification**. To be justified is to be seen by God as righteous, despite our sin, because of Christ's cleansing work on the cross.

➤ As a child, you may have learned that justification means "just as if I never sinned." What does justification mean to you as an adult?

➤ Justification is a one-time event. According to Romans 10:9-10, when are we justified?

The moment we are justified by our faith in Jesus Christ, we begin the lifelong journey of becoming more like Him. **Sanctification** is this process of becoming holy and set apart for God. Our purification is not complete until the day we are taken home in glory.

Many Christians confuse justification and sanctification; as a result, they fear losing their salvation during the purification process. There is no way we could persevere to the end in our own strength and power, but praise God, Jesus Christ has the power to keep us from falling. He will present us before God's glorious throne without fault. Romans 8:30 assures us that if we have been justified we *will* be glorified!

➤ In John 17:17-19, Jesus prayed that His disciples would be sanctified by the truth. His prayer also reveals what truth is. According to John 17:17, what is truth?

➤ How is acknowledging the truth of God's Word part of your sanctification process?

Your participation in the First Place program is also part of your sanctification. You acknowledge God's truth through keeping the Nine Commitments.

➤ What truth do you need to embrace right now so that you can complete today's segment of your journey toward Christlike wholeness?

Though we have the privilege and the responsibility to give God glory every day of our Christian life, **glorification**, like justification, is also a one-time event.

➤ Read 2 Thessalonians 1:5-10. When are we glorified?

➤ Romans 8:30 gives us a guarantee with regard to our glorification. What awesome promise is contained in that verse?

 Father, thank You for giving me Your Word, which is truth [see John 17:17].

Father God, as I journey toward You in the footsteps of Your Son, under the power and guidance of Your Holy Spirit, help me to always tell myself the truth so that I can worship You in spirit and in truth [see John 4:24].

DAY 6: *Reflections*

When Jesus went into the wilderness, His knowledge of the Word of God was all He took with Him. Jesus knew His Father's words were His most valuable survival tool as He faced a time of temptation that could have derailed His whole life purpose. Jesus did not have to take a bunch of large scrolls out into the desert with Him. All the Scriptures He needed to counter the enemy's attacks were in His head and in His heart. Jesus knew there would not be enough time to roll and unroll scrolls while the enemy was tempting Him! There would be no time to fumble around for just the right verse, and relying on a loose paraphrase would leave out valuable portions of the truth. Jesus internally carried the Word, exactly as it was written, with Him wherever He went so that He could readily counter Satan at any moment.

As we saw in this week's study, God's Word is truth—truth that can set us free. Our responsibility is to learn the truth so that we can apply it to our life situations with accuracy. Memorizing God's Word is one of the

Nine Commitments of First Place, but Scripture memorization is more than just a First Place commitment. It is vital to our survival when we encounter distortion, denial, delusion and the devil's many disguises.

God promises never to tempt us beyond what we can bear, and He tells us we will always be given an escape route when the tempter invites us to satisfy a legitimate need through an illegitimate means (see 1 Corinthians 10:13). Often that escape route is through the wisdom of Scripture verses that we have memorized. The memory verses of First Place are specifically selected for the battle we must fight as we strive to honor God by caring for our bodies. Each memory verse is also anchored to the week's lesson so that when we recall the verse, we will also recall the truths we learned in that week's study. By memorizing 10 Scriptures in the course of each Bible study, we will soon have a storehouse of verses and lessons to strengthen us when we find ourselves in perilous situations in which we must counter the evil one with the exact truth of God's Word. Through faithful memorization, we will always find grace to help us in our time of need (see Hebrews 4:16).

Praise be to You, O Lord! Teach me Your decrees so that with my lips I can recount all the laws that come from Your mouth. I have hidden Your word in my heart, so I will not sin against You [see Psalm 119:11-12].

Sovereign Lord, I will keep my way pure by living according to the truth of Your Word [see Psalm 119:9].

Father, thank You for sending the Holy Spirit to guide me into all truth and to remind me of everything You have said to me [see John 14:26].

DAY 7: *Reflections*

This week's lessons have focused on the truth and our need to know the truth as it is written in the Bible. There is also another truth we must always tell ourselves if we are going to allow the truth to set us free. We need to be honest with ourselves about our circumstances and motivations. Until we are honest with ourselves, we will not see our need to cry out to God for mercy and grace.

Psalm 107 is a wonderful reminder of the connection between crying to the Lord in our distress and receiving grace and help in our time of need. Throughout this psalm we read of God's people in perilous situations— some of their own making! They were hungry and thirsty, and their lives faded away (v. 5); they were oppressed by bitter labor, but they had no one to help them when they stumbled (v. 12). They were in darkness and deep gloom (v. 14); they suffered affliction and were near the gates of death (v. 18). They were at their wits' end (v. 27)! In the midst of such misery, they did the only thing they could do: "They cried to the Lord in their trouble, and he delivered them from their distress" (vv. 6,13,19). Verse 20 reveals how God delivered them: "He sent forth his word and healed them." That same deliverance is available to us too. No matter how dire our situation, crying out to the Lord brings relief. God is always attentive to the heartfelt cries of His suffering people.

All positive change begins with awareness, and awareness involves telling yourself the truth—no matter how painful it is to do so. Then when you earnestly cry out to the Lord for relief, He will come to your assistance. He will always send forth His healing Word, but He waits for you to ask for His help before He intervenes.

Without healthy boundaries we will continue to fall prey to the enemy's wiles. God longs to repair our broken lives, restore our integrity and allow us to reclaim our heritage as His dearly beloved children. In the weeks ahead, we will begin the boundary-rebuilding process. Today, through the words of Psalm 107, let us find courage to begin the work, confident that the Lord is ready to help us when we cry out to Him.

The words of the prophet Isaiah assure us that God longs to be gracious to us. He rises to show us compassion. We will weep no more because our God will be gracious when we cry for help (see Isaiah 30:18-19). "As soon as he hears, he will answer you" (Isaiah 30:19).

 Lord God Almighty, You are worthy of thanks and praise. I will call to You in my distress and I will be saved from my enemies [see Psalm 18:3].

Merciful and compassionate Lord, when I cry to You in my trouble, I can rest assured that You will send forth Your Word and heal me [see Psalm 107:19-20].

Father, Your Word is truth. Jesus, You came so that I can know the truth and be free from the tyranny of sin. Holy Spirit, You are my counselor and my guide as I begin the rebuilding process. When I am afraid, I will trust in my almighty God.

GROUP PRAYER REQUESTS TODAY'S DATE:_____

NAME	REQUEST	RESULTS

RESPOND TO THE CALL

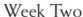
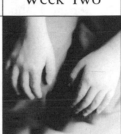

MEMORY VERSE
*Surely the arm of the LORD is not too short to save,
nor his ear too dull to hear.*
Isaiah 59:1

Nehemiah was a brilliant administrator called by God to rebuild the crumbled walls around Jerusalem so that God's people could live in safety. Much like walls and gates surround a city to protect its citizens from intruders, our personal boundaries allow us to live productive lives free from the threat of unwanted intrusion. Our boundaries define us, and, like physical property lines, they tell us where we stop and where others begin. Boundaries determine what we are responsible to maintain and what things others are responsible to maintain.

By giving us a detailed account of how Nehemiah rebuilt the broken walls around Jerusalem, God has graciously given us a template to use when our personal boundaries need restoration so that we can keep out intruders that threaten to invade and hinder our growth. Just as God called Nehemiah to undertake the rebuilding process, so He calls us to restore our damaged boundaries—both external and internal so that we can worship Him with single-minded devotion.

DAY 1: *Hear the Truth*

Matthew 11:15 says, "He who has ears, let him hear." Not only does Jesus exhort His followers to speak the truth, but we must also be willing to *listen* to the truth. And like telling the truth, listening to the truth is often painful.

Between 605 and 586 b.c., God used the Babylonians to mete out His judgment on the Israelites in Judah and on the holy city of Jerusalem. Much of the nation was taken into captivity in Babylon, including Nehemiah. We begin Nehemiah's story years later, when he received word about his countrymen who were left in Judah.

❧ Read Nehemiah 1:1-3. What did the visitors from Judah tell Nehemiah about the Jewish remnant that survived the exile?

❧ Why do you think broken walls and burned gates would be a problem for the remnant people living in Jerusalem?

❧ Nehemiah heard the report and accepted it as accurate. What do you think would have happened if Nehemiah had denied or discounted the facts he heard about the plight of God's people in Jerusalem?

We learned about denial in last week's lesson. **Minimizing** and **exaggerating** the truth are just as dangerous as flat-out denial. Minimizing the truth is downplaying the facts so that we do not have to acknowledge the severity of the problem. Exaggerating the truth means making things out to be much worse than they really are.

Satan uses all three weapons—denial, minimization and exaggeration—to keep us from hearing the truth that can set us free.

❧ What truth are you denying about your current situation that keeps you from taking appropriate action to remedy the problem?

≫ What health-related concerns are you minimizing so that you won't have to face a painful reality?

It is easy to exaggerate our real problems in an attempt to get extra attention, sympathy or pity. Some of us have been exaggerating for so long, we no longer even recognize when we twist the truth in this manner.

≫ How has exaggeration kept you from coming up with an effective solution to your genuine distress?

≫ Turn to Revelation 3:14. How did Jesus describe Himself as He addressed the church at Laodicea?

How can you be this type of witness when assessing the condition of your life?

Father, I thank You that I can face the truth, no matter how painful, because I am confident that You will never leave me to face my troubles alone.

God of truth and love, help me to never deny, minimize or exaggerate my problems. When I tell the truth about my situation, I can approach Your throne of grace with confidence and receive help in my time of need [see Hebrews 4:16].

DAY 2: *Pray Without Ceasing*

"Well, I've done all I can do. All I can do now is pray," are words we hear all too often from the lips of God's people. We worry and we fret and we ring our hands in anguish, and when all else fails, we finally ask for God's help. First Thessalonians 5:17 commands us to "pray continually," yet most of us use prayer as our last resort, not our first line of defense.

Let's pick up where we left off in the book of Nehemiah to learn an important lesson about prayer.

≫ Read Nehemiah 1:4-11. What was the first thing Nehemiah did when he heard the distressing report?

Nehemiah did not immediately swing into action! He sat down and wept. He spent days mourning, fasting and praying before God.

≫ How do you usually react when you receive bad news?

- ❏ Call my friends and complain
- ❏ Deny, minimize or exaggerate the truth
- ❏ Eat
- ❏ Feel sorry for myself
- ❏ Find a project to keep me busy
- ❏ Get angry and blame others for the problem
- ❏ Get discouraged and depressed
- ❏ Go shopping
- ❏ Panic
- ❏ Pray for God's help and guidance

By studying Nehemiah's prayer (Nehemiah 1:5-11) we can learn how to bring our heartfelt sorrows to the Lord. List the verses and the key words Nehemiah used for each element of effective prayer. An example has been given.

Element	Verse(s)	Key Words
Praise	5	*God of heaven; great and awesome*
Supplication		
Confession		
Recall Promises		
Rededication		
Requests		

➤ How can studying Nehemiah's reaction to the devastating news of Jerusalem help you in times of bad tidings?

➤ What did you learn from today's lesson that you can apply to the First Place Prayer commitment?

Pray that the Holy Spirit will help you apply these truths the next time you are confronted with disturbing news.

 O Lord, God of heaven, let Your ear be attentive to my prayer, for I delight in revering Your name [see Nehemiah 1:11].
Father, I claim Your precious promises of reconciliation and restoration through the redeeming work of Jesus Christ, applied to my life through the Holy Spirit's power.

DAY 3: *Pave the Pathway with Prayer*

Throughout our entire study of Nehemiah's rebuilding project, we will see Nehemiah repeat the same pattern over and over: prayer before planning, planning before action and action that leads back to prayer. Prayer preceded every action Nehemiah took. With careful observation and discipline, we can learn to use the same cycle in our boundary-rebuilding efforts.

Using the elements in Nehemiah's prayer we identified yesterday, today we will build our own lament. The elements are listed below. Use them to construct your own words in a heartfelt prayer to the God of heaven, the great and awesome God who keeps His covenant of love with those who love Him and obey His commands. Under the rededication section, rededicate your participation in First Place. If you need more space, you can continue your prayer in your journal.

Praise—

Supplication—

Confession—

Recall Promises—

Rededication—

Requests—

※ Nehemiah 1:5,9-10 gives us valuable information about those with whom God keeps covenants (promises). What do these verses tell us?

※ Are you participating in First Place in a way that merits God's blessing?

What do you need to change in order to return to God and obey His commands as a prelude to success?

 You are forgiving and good, O Lord, abounding in love to all who call to you. Hear my prayer, O Lord; listen to my cry for mercy. In the day of my trouble I will call to you, for you will answer me [Psalm 86:5-7].

DAY 4: *Formulate a Plan*

As a result of his prayer, Nehemiah was able to come up with a plan. Just as we gleaned valuable insight from Nehemiah's prayer, we can also draw on his administrative skills as we begin to formulate our own rebuilding plan. Take time now to prayerfully read Nehemiah 2:1-9.

Because we do not speak Hebrew, most of us miss two important dates recorded in the first two chapters of Nehemiah. Nehemiah 1:1 tells us the visitors brought the bad news to Nehemiah in Kislev, which is the ninth month of the Jewish calendar. Nisan (see Nehemiah 2:1) is the first month of the Jewish year.

➣ How long did Nehemiah pray and plan before taking action?

What can we learn from these dates about waiting patiently in prayer for God's timing?

➣ How did God use Nehemiah's occupation to present his question before King Artaxerxes (1:11—2:1)?

Our God works through circumstances. Romans 8:28 declares, "In all things God works for the good of those who love him." Even the timing of the arrival of the wine to be brought before the king was part of God's plan for Nehemiah's success!

➣ What circumstances might God be using in your life to tell you the time is right to begin rebuilding your broken boundaries?

Read Nehemiah 2:2-3, noting Nehemiah's emotions as he went before the king. Even though Nehemiah was afraid, he drew his boldness from his relationship with God. That same humble boldness is available to all who call on God and allow Him to be their strength.

➣ How can humble boldness help you succeed in First Place?

When the king asked Nehemiah what he wanted, Nehemiah had a ready answer. His prayer had allowed him to formulate a plan that included four things. Look at the verses listed below and list those four things.

Verse 5—

Verse 6—

Verse 7—

Verse 8—

≫ Why did the king grant Nehemiah's requests (v. 8)?

≫ Verse 9 tells us Nehemiah got one thing he did not ask for. What unexpected blessing did Nehemiah receive from the king?

God's gracious hand is also on you. Place yourself before your King and ask Him for the things you need to begin the work before you, confident that you will get even more than you ask for or can even imagine. Write your prayer in the space provided or in your journal.

Gracious Lord, thank You for Your lavish love. You always do immeasurably more than I can ask for or imagine when I put my trust in You [see Ephesians 3:20].
Remember me with favor, O my God [Nehemiah 13:31].

DAY 5: *Be Response-Able*

Often we hear and acknowledge bad news, but then we immediately turn the energy we could use to respond appropriately into anger and blame. Instead of taking our complaints to God, we lash out at or burden others— often those who are not willing to be part of positive change. When we begin looking at our brokenness, we easily start blaming others for our distress.

➴ What motivated Nehemiah's prayer and humble boldness (1:1-3; 2:3,10)?

Although Nehemiah was not to blame for the great trouble and distress of God's people, he was willing to take appropriate action.

➴ What can we learn from Nehemiah about blame and responsibility?

Some of us have been badly damaged by unfortunate circumstances beyond our control. We are not responsible for the damage, but we are responsible for praying, planning and taking appropriate action.

➴ What does Romans 12:19-21 tell us about seeking revenge on those whom we feel have injured us?

When we leave revenge to God, we are free to take positive action. That is how we are able to overcome evil with good.

➴ Make a list of the people whom you feel have injured you.

As one forgiven by God, you are called to forgive everyone on that list. Forgiveness is a conscious decision. Write out a prayer to God, giving Him permission to deal with each person on that list as He sees fit. Be careful not to tell God what you think He should do. Just lay the wrongs at the foot of the Cross and walk away.

Now that you aren't hindered by the need for revenge, you can take responsible action. Divide the word "responsible" into two words: "response" and "able." We are able to do all things through Christ who gives us strength (see Philippians 4:13). In Christ's strength, we are always able to respond in appropriate ways that give glory and honor to our King.

➣ List one appropriate action you need to take in order to move on from the feelings of revenge or other negative feelings you have been harboring against the people who have injured you.

Now determine to be response-able and follow through with that action; you are able to do all things through Christ, who gives you strength.

Compassionate and merciful God, I will forgive those who have hurt me because You have forgiven me and I want to follow Your example [see Colossians 3:13].

My Lord and my God, help me not to be overcome by evil, but to overcome evil with good [see Romans 12:21].

DAY 6: *Reflections*

Most Bible scholars rely on a principle called "the law of first reference" when interpreting the correct meaning of Scripture. This law states that the first use of a word or phrase spoken by God sets the stage for the underlying meaning of that word or phrase throughout the remainder of Scripture. For example, the earliest mention of the arm of God appears in Exodus 6:6-7.

> Say to the Israelites: "I am the Lord, and I will bring you out from under the yoke of the Egyptians. I will free you from being slaves to them, and I will redeem you with an outstretched arm and with mighty acts of judgment. I will take you as my own people, and I will be your God. Then you will know that I am the Lord your God, who brought you out from under the yoke of the Egyptians."

From that point on, God's outstretched arm is symbolic of the awesome power of God as He delivers His people from oppression and slavery. Numbers 11:23, Deuteronomy 4:34, Jeremiah 27:5 and Psalm 44:3 also refer to the delivering power of God's outstretched arm. Take time now to read and reflect on these verses.

Now recall this week's memory verse, a powerful reminder of both God's awesome power and His tender loving care of His faithful children. When Isaiah said, "Surely the arm of the Lord is not too short to save, nor his ear too dull to hear," he was encouraging God's people to remember how Jehovah saved them from oppression and slavery because He cared enough to hear their cries and take powerful action to deliver them.

If you are struggling with oppression and slavery to sin, be encouraged and strengthened by these verses that speak of "the arm of God." Put them on index cards and read them often. Hide them in your heart and mind so that when trouble comes you will not be tempted to deny, minimize or exaggerate the truth. You will not fall back into destructive behaviors if you go before God with humble boldness and rely on His mighty strength to shore up your weaknesses. Cry out to Him. Claim His promises. Confess your sins. Praise Him for His compassionate power. Rededicate yourself to Him—and then wait expectantly for your deliverance. Take heart, dear child of God. "The arm of the Lord is not too short to save, nor his ear too dull to hear." He will show Himself mighty to save!

Great and awesome God, let Your ears be attentive and Your eyes open to hear the prayer I offer to You today [see Nehemiah 1:6].

Lord, You are my portion; therefore, I will wait for You. Your compassions never fail; they are new every morning. You are so faithful to me [see Lamentations 3:22-24].

I will put my hope in You, O Lord, both now and forevermore [see Psalm 131:3].

DAY 7: *Reflections*

In the face of forces that threaten our well-being, we often do not know what to do. This week we have seen how Nehemiah responded when given distressing news about the remnant people who had returned from exile. When he didn't know what to do, Nehemiah prayed, confident that God would hear his prayer and come to the aid of His covenant people.

Jehoshaphat, another leader appointed by God, also responded to bad tidings by seeking help from the Lord.

If calamity comes upon us, whether the sword of judgment, or plague or famine, we will stand in your presence before this temple that bears your Name and will cry out to you in our distress, and you will hear us and save us. We have no power to face this vast army that is attacking us. We do not know what to do, but our eyes are upon you (2 Chronicles 20:9,12).

In the face of seeming disaster, Jehoshaphat confidently responded by focusing his attention on God rather than on the impending doom. Instead of relying on our own reasoning ability, our first responsibility is to rely on God. When crises come, our priority must be to let God be God.

When we choose to focus our thoughts on God and acknowledge His might and power, He hears our cries and shows Himself mighty to save. When we turn to God in our utter helplessness, we will always hear Him say, "Don't be afraid or discouraged, for this battle is not yours but God's. Take your position, stand firm and see the deliverance the Lord will give you" (see 2 Chronicles 20:15-17).

O Lord, "We do not know what to do, but our eyes are upon you" (2 Chronicles 20:12). God's people are always able to respond by putting their hope and trust in the One who has promised to be their strength in times of trouble.

Sovereign Lord, thank You that when I cry out to You, You show me great and unsearchable things that I do not know [see Jeremiah 33:3].

You, O Lord, will keep me in perfect peace. My mind is steadfast, because I trust in You [see Isaiah 26:3].

Father, I know Your arm is not too short to save, and Your ears are not too dull to hear. When I am afraid, I will trust in You [see Isaiah 59:1]

GROUP PRAYER REQUESTS   TODAY'S DATE:_____

NAME	REQUEST	RESULTS

ASSESS
THE DAMAGE

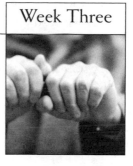

MEMORY VERSE
*Like a city whose walls are broken down is a man
who lacks self-control.*
Proverbs 25:28

Perhaps you have been wondering what rebuilding your personal boundaries has to do with success in the First Place program. This week's memory
verse contains the answer to that question: Our internal walls are broken
down due to a lack of self-control. No matter how diligent our efforts, we
are doomed to fail unless we are able to control what goes into and comes
out of our personal space. This is why recognizing and restoring our crumbled inner walls is so important to our success in First Place. Until we have
rebuilt our boundaries, uncontrollable forces will continue to sabotage our
plans and leave us living in fear and defeat

> Note: Before you begin week three, complete Wellness
> Worksheet One (pages 155-163), which explains physical,
> mental, emotional and spiritual boundaries and will help you
> make a thorough assessment of your internal protection system.

DAY 1: *A Private Inspection*

With God's protection and provision Nehemiah arrived safely in Jerusalem. Messengers had told Nehemiah about the damage and ruin. God
had put it on Nehemiah's heart to rebuild the walls; however, Nehemiah
knew that before he could finalize his plans he had to know firsthand the
extent of the damage.

Our government officials do the same thing today. In the wake of calamity, they personally tour the damaged area so that they can accurately assess the extent of the devastation.

Please read Nehemiah 2:11—16, and then answer the following questions:

➣ When did Nehemiah conduct his initial assessment of the damaged walls?

➣ Who did Nehemiah take with him on his secret mission?

Private planning always comes before public victory. Nehemiah knew he should have his inner plans in place before he revealed them publicly.

➣ Why is private planning important in your own boundary-rebuilding project?

Later this week we will look at a group of folks who were angry because someone was coming to help the Israelites in their distress (see Nehemiah 2:10). They saw Nehemiah as a threat to their position and power. You too may encounter people who will feel threatened when they learn you are going to take steps to rebuild your life.

➣ What could happen to your plans if you make them public too soon?

⤳ What valuable lessons can you learn from Nehemiah's nighttime assessment that will help you achieve ultimate success in First Place through your boundary-rebuilding project?

Call a member of your First Place group today and ask him or her to be part of your inner circle as you examine the broken walls that produce fear, defeat and frustration in your attempt to achieve steady weight loss through the First Place program.

Loving Father, thank You for putting on my heart the work of repairing my inner protection system so that I can live a life characterized by self control.

Your love, O Lord, endures forever. Thank You for the assurance that You will never abandon the work of Your hands [see Psalm 138:8].

DAY 2: Walls and Gates

Protective walls of stone equipped with gates that were often guarded by armed sentinels surrounded ancient cities, providing protection and security for those living within. From the top of these walls, watchmen would survey the countryside, scanning the horizon for signs of approaching visitors—and invaders. These watchmen determined who was allowed to enter the city and when the gates needed to be closed to protect the city's residents. In the morning the town's elders would gather at the city gates to negotiate business transactions and debate civic affairs.

Strong walls and trustworthy sentinels allowed residents to carry on the business of living in a safe and productive manner. Without secure walls and well-guarded gates, the people would have lived in constant chaos and anxiety.

Likewise, our personal boundaries let in the good things needed for life and health, and keep out what is toxic, harmful and life threatening. Well-maintained inner walls and gates allow us to share our inner goodness with others. They also allow us to safely dispose of the things that threaten to pollute our private space.

Nehemiah 3 outlines the repair process, including a list of the gates and who rebuilt them. List the gates in the spaces provided below. To the right of each gate name, write a brief description of why you think that gate was important to the safety, security and commerce of the city.

Gate   Purpose

_____   _____

_____   _____

_____   _____

_____   _____

_____   _____

_____   _____

_____   _____

_____   _____

_____   _____

The gates allowed the townsfolk to bring in supplies, muster their troops, care for their animals, engage in commerce, travel to foreign cities, dispose of refuse, practice personal hygiene and bury their dead.

What would happen to a city without intact walls?

What would happen if a city had fortified walls but no gates?

What is located inside the most fortified part of the city walls?

Read 1 Corinthians 6:19. Based on your answer to the previous question, why is it so important to protect and care for our bodies?

 What have you learned today that helps you understand the correlation between broken-down walls in a city and broken internal boundaries? What have you learned about self-control?

How can you personally apply this insight in order to succeed in the First Place program?

 Gracious God, thank You for establishing boundaries for my protection and provision.

God Almighty, You call me to be self-controlled and alert so that I can pray [see 1 Peter 4:7]. Help me build healthy boundaries that allow me to be obedient to Your commands.

DAY 3: *An Accurate Report*

When Nehemiah had completed his tour of the damaged walls and gates, he went to the people and gave them a type of State of the Union address.

 According to Nehemiah 2:17, what did Nehemiah tell the people?

In Jeremiah 6:14-15 we read about false prophets who proclaimed peace when there was no peace. Read this passage before answering the following questions.

≫ What would have happened to the people if Nehemiah had distorted the facts and led them to believe things were okay when they were not?

Drawing from what you learned in weeks one and two, why was it important that Nehemiah presented the facts without denying, distorting, minimizing or exaggerating the truth?

Not only did Nehemiah give an accurate report, but he also gave the reason for undertaking the rebuilding project.

≫ Look again at Nehemiah 2:17. What reason did Nehemiah give the Jews for needing to rebuild the wall?

How do your broken boundary walls leave you living a life of disgrace?

If you have not done so already, complete "Assessing Your Boundaries" in Wellness Worksheet One (pages 155-163). You will present your State of the Union report at your First Place meeting this week.

≫ What small step are you prepared to take today to make your plan become reality?

Sovereign Lord, I am thankful that I can tell the truth about the condition of my life because I know You accept me just as I am today and will never turn Your back on me, no matter how desperate my situation.

Father, I thank You for the assurance that when I commit my plans to You, they will succeed [see Proverbs 16:3].

DAY 4: *Encouraging Words*

In addition to giving an accurate report, Nehemiah included words of encouragement when he addressed the people. Nehemiah told the people two important facts that caused them to respond favorably to the restoration plan (see Nehemiah 2:18).

Recall from weeks one and two:

- The gracious hand of God was upon Nehemiah.
- The king confirmed Nehemiah's plan and made his journey to Jerusalem possible.

≫ How was God's gracious hand on you when He called you to join First Place? Include the circumstances of your life and the messengers He sent to you as part of His plan.

≫ What things did others do and say to confirm God's plan and purpose for your work once God had laid the rebuilding project on your heart (e.g., special help you may have received that made First Place attendance possible)?

❧ Nehemiah's words encouraged the people to reply, "Let us start rebuilding" (v. 18). How do the events leading up to this Bible study encourage you to start this good work and confirm God's plan for you?

❧ Philippians 1:6 reminds us that God assures the success of our rebuilding projects. According to this verse, when will the project be complete?

❧ Why is the First Place Scripture memory commitment an essential part of your rebuilding efforts?

❧ Which Scripture memory verses will you use to encourage yourself and others as you begin your personal restoration project?

Write a note to someone in your First Place group today. Include encouragement from God's Word and assurance that victory is certain because God will see his or her good work to completion.

Lord God Almighty, I trust in You. I am confident You will bring the good work You have started in me to victorious completion [see Philippians 1:6].

Father, today my heart is full of gratitude and love as I recall how Your gracious hand has provided me with everything I need to complete the work You have placed before me.

DAY 5: *Answers for the Opposition*

Unfortunately, not everyone who hears about our rebuilding projects will be enthusiastic and supportive. There may be some people who oppose our efforts because they feel their positions and security are threatened.

Nehemiah 2:10 introduces us to a group of men who were disturbed when they heard that someone had come to promote the welfare of the Israelites. Throughout our study we will see how these subversive leaders tried to undermine Nehemiah's work and fill the people with fear and discouragement. Whenever we begin a rebuilding project, we can also expect opposition. Part of our rebuilding plan must include identifying the enemy and finding appropriate ways to defend ourselves.

>>- What did some of the officials do when they heard about Nehemiah's plans (2:19)?

There may be those who mock and ridicule your boundary rebuilding efforts. Some of your opposition may be silent or passive-aggressive, but just because these people are not openly hostile does not mean the opposition does not exist.

>>- Who are the naysayers (well-intentioned or otherwise) in your life who will try to thwart your plans and keep you in defeat and despair? Beside each name, write the reason you feel they will not be supportive of your boundary-rebuilding endeavors (e.g., jealousy, fear, pride, a need for power and control).

>>- Carefully read Nehemiah's response to those who mocked him. How did he respond to their jeers (2:20)?

➤ Acts 4:1-22 tells us about two other men who exhibited humble boldness in the face of strong opposition. Who are these men and what was their response to those who tried to stop their mission (vv. 19-20)?

➤ Whom are you pleasing when you begin caring for your body and restoring the broken inner walls that shame you?

Is pleasing God more important to you than pleasing the men and women who oppose you, or are you still more interested in gaining human approval? Explain your answer.

➤ Share a time this past week when you chose to please people rather than God.

➤ Read Colossians 4:5-6. Why do you think it is important that we know how to answer everyone, even those who oppose our faith?

Nehemiah was confident that the God of heaven would give him success. We also need to be confident in God's ability to ensure our victory in First Place.

≫ How will you reply to those who oppose your efforts to honor God through repairing the broken walls that keep you living in disgrace?

God of heaven and Earth, thank You for giving me success when I undertake Your work and obey Your Word in the strength of Your might and power.

May the words of my mouth and the meditation of my heart be pleasing in your sight, O Lord, my Rock and my Redeemer [Psalm 19:14].

DAY 6: *Reflections*

Boundaries are part of God's creation order and therefore part of His plan and purpose for our lives. Genesis 1:2 tells us that the earth was originally formless, empty and covered with darkness. The Spirit of God hovered over the waters and established boundaries that gave God's emerging creation form and definition: light and darkness, land and sea, earth and sky—each with its own boundaries and purpose in God's newly formed world. As creation progressed, vegetation and living creatures were created—also defined by God-given boundaries and purpose. Finally, man was created, and he too was defined by his boundaries.

In addition to physical form, humankind was given boundary limitations in the form of God's righteous laws and decrees. Though these boundaries are not visible, as are riverbanks, tree bark and skin, our internal boundaries also protect us. Our internal boundaries define who we are, what we stand for and to whom we belong. Just as a stream without banks quickly becomes a puddle, people without boundaries quickly lose their uniqueness and definition. As often as we resist our God-given limitations, God repeatedly tells us that His boundaries define us as His people and put us in right relationship with Him.

This week we looked at the correlation between damaged boundaries and lack of self-control. Self-control is essential to success in the First

Place program. Take a moment to remember a time when your life spun out of control because you could not say no to someone's requests. Instead of being defined by God's purpose for your life, you took on someone else's agenda. Spend some time reflecting on the purpose of boundaries in your life, and prayerfully determine once again to restore your broken walls and burned gates so that you can live a victorious life that gives glory to God and manifests His presence in every aspect of your being.

 Sovereign Lord, from the beginning You have established boundaries that give Your creation purpose and definition. Help me to honor what You have created and called good.

Almighty Father, I desire to be transformed by the renewing of my mind. Please send Your Holy Spirit to hover over me and bring light to my darkness and clarity to my confusion.

O Lord my God, I take refuge in You; save and deliver me from those who attempt to thwart my plans and keep me from reclaiming my heritage as Your child [see Psalm 7:1].

DAY 7: *Reflections*

Take a few moments to reflect on what you have learned in the first three weeks of this Bible study. If you are not already keeping a spiritual prayer journal, now is the time to begin. Here are some ideas to get you started:

- Write down the important lessons you have gleaned from your studies thus far.
- Commit to God those steps you have determined you must take in the days ahead.
- Pay close attention to the ways God has brought you to this place and time.
- Thank Him for His Word and for His promises that will sustain you in the days ahead.
- Jot down the First Place memory verses that will become part of your rebuilding process, and refer to them often.
- Record the names of those in your inner circle who can help you plan privately, laying the foundation for public victory.

- Thank God for giving you a First Place group in which you can find safety and security until your own inner walls are strong enough to keep out invaders.
- Write down the names of those who may oppose your efforts and begin praying that God will deliver you from people who would like to persuade you that there is no help for you in God.

Nehemiah 3 gives a detailed account of the rebuilding process as the Israelites worked together to rebuild the broken walls and gates. Make your prayer journal your personal, detailed account of your rebuilding process. Like a captain accurately maintains a log during a long voyage, take time each evening to record the day's important events on the pages of your journal. Include dates so that you will be able to recount your progress during the victory celebration that will come at the end of this study.

 I praise You, O Lord, for You are my rock, my loving God, my fortress, my stronghold and my deliverer [see Psalm 144:1-2].

My soul praises You, O Lord. I will praise You all my life; I will sing praises to Your name as long as I live [see Psalm 146:1-2].

Merciful God, I will sing of Your great love forever; with my mouth I will make Your faithfulness known [see Psalm 89:1].

GROUP PRAYER REQUESTS   TODAY'S DATE:_____

NAME	REQUEST	RESULTS

REVEAL FALSE BOUNDARIES

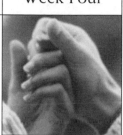

MEMORY VERSE

But you are a shield around me, O Lord;
you bestow glory on me and lift up my head.
Psalm 3:3

Many of us have damaged personal boundaries. As a result, we do not know where we stop and where others begin. We take on others' responsibilities and allow invaders to come into our personal space unhindered. Often, in a self-defeating attempt to protect ourselves, we build flimsy false boundaries to replace our crumbled internal walls.

When our internal protection system is damaged, food often becomes one of our false boundaries. We avoid intimacy—which would make us vulnerable to being taken advantage of again—by gaining weight and becoming less attractive. The "comfort" of food is less scary than the prospect of real relationships in which we would be forced to rebuild boundaries to protect us from further abuse.

Food is not the only false boundary we rely on as we try to find the safety and security missing from our inner world. Anger, deception, possessions, prestige, compulsive busyness and the need to control others are some of the other false boundaries to which we cling.

This week we will observe how the things we cling to in a futile effort to feel safe actually become our idols. Instead of being part of the solution, they only compound the problem and push us further into defeat and despair. The world offers many forms of temporary relief, but only reliance on God can give us true and lasting security.

DAY 1: *Our Safety and Security*

Throughout Scripture God presents Himself as our protector and defender. He wants to be the One to whom we cling when we are insecure and afraid. Yet much like small children cling to security blankets and teddy bears when Mom and Dad aren't around, as adults we latch on to other things when our security is threatened. Though now we can easily see that blankets and toys are only illusions of security, we are blinded to those things we hold on to instead of allowing God to be our shield.

David wrote many of his psalms while he was fleeing from his enemies. Psalm 18 is the song of praise David sang after God delivered him from the hand of Saul.

➤ Read Psalm 18:1-6 and list the ways David described God in this hymn of praise.

➤ Recall a time this week when God was your rock, the One you ran to for safety and security. As you recount, be sure to thank Him for being your refuge in time of trouble.

In Psalm 3:3, our memory verse, David described God as our shield. Take a moment to read all of Psalm 3 so that you can put verse 3 in proper perspective, and then answer the following questions:

➤ What was David's dilemma (v. 1)?

➤ What were David's foes saying to him (v. 2)?

➤ Why was David confident in the face of opposition (v. 3)?

➤ To whom did David cry out (v. 4)?

➤ As a result of David's trust in God, what could he do (v. 5)?

➤ Who sustained David during his trials (v. 5)?

➤ What was David's boast (v. 8)?

The Bible becomes more real to us when we put ourselves in the scene instead of reading Scripture as a story about someone else. Take the questions above and substitute your name for David's.

➤ What is my dilemma?

≫ What are my foes saying to me?

≫ Am I crying out to God in confidence, or am I putting my trust in other things?

≫ Does my trust in God allow me to lie down and sleep peacefully?

≫ Who is sustaining me during my present trial?

≫ What is my boast?

Take your words and write them into a song of praise to God, the One who lifts up your head. If you have been trusting in something other than God to sustain you, affirm your future trust in God.

Mighty God, You are my fortress. You are alive! You are my rock, and I will exalt You O God, my Savior [see Psalm 18:46].

I love you, O Lord, my strength [Psalm 18:1].

DAY 2: *Our Rock*

At the end of yesterday's lesson you wrote a personal song of praise to God, your shield and the One who lifts up your head. Before you begin today's lesson, reread your psalm and thank God for being your rock.

Now turn to Isaiah 44:6-8 and read how God describes Himself to His covenant people. In verse 8 God poses two questions. Using God's own Words, answer Him.

➤ What did God proclaim long ago (v. 6)?

➤ Is there any God besides the Lord Almighty (v. 8)?

Repeat these affirmations throughout the day.

Speaking through the prophet Isaiah, God went on to describe the folly of those who bow down to idols.

➤ Read Isaiah 44:17-20. Summarize what God has to say about idols in this passage.

What does the idol worshiper say as he bows down to the block of wood (v. 17)?

≫ In the end, what are those who worship idols prevented from realizing (v. 20)?

≫ According to Isaiah 43:11, who does God say is the only One who can save us?

≫ After reading Habakkuk 2:18, rewrite the passage in your own words.

Anything apart from God that we look to for protection, security and safety is every bit as much an idol as the block of wood Isaiah described. All that has changed throughout the centuries is the object of our idol worship. We may not carve idols out of wood, but we have substituted other things for the God who commands us to have no other gods before Him (see Exodus 20:3).

As we conclude today's lesson, read and reflect on the words of Isaiah 44:22. Take time to thank God for sweeping away your offenses like the morning mist. All of us have turned to other gods in a desperate attempt to feel secure, but God has redeemed us from our bondage.

Almighty God, I humbly acknowledge that You are the Lord; apart from you there is no Savior [see Isaiah 43:11].

My Lord and my God, I confess my sins before You. I have looked to other gods for safety and security, and foolishly trusted in idols of my own making. Thank You for Your promise of forgiveness and restoration through the precious blood of Jesus, shed for me.

DAY 3: *Our Real Enemy*

As we've already learned, Satan will do everything in his power to undermine the rebuilding process to which God has called us. The words of the apostle Paul in Ephesians 6:12 remind us that our battle is fought in the spiritual realms. We fight an unseen enemy.

≫ Summarize Ephesians 6:12 in your own words.

≫ David correctly identified his many foes in Psalm 3. According to verse 2, what did his enemies say to David?

No matter what form or shape our opponents take in the physical world, the real enemy is the voice that tells us, "God will not deliver you."

≫ Exodus 17:1-7 gives us added insight into where the voice of the real enemy often resides. When faced with a trial, what did the Israelites do and say?

The Israelites themselves questioned God's presence and His ability to provide for their needs. We all have negative voices inside our minds too. When faced with trials and temptations, we question God's promises. The voices inside us try to convince us that God will not deliver us. Many of these negative voices are the result of childhood trauma. As children we did not understand the implications of evil and sin and spiritual warfare.

When bad things happened to us, we came to the erroneous conclusion that God did not love us and would not protect us. Part of Christian maturity includes learning to challenge the negative voices that have dominated our thought process and convinced us God will not deliver us.

➢ What did the apostle Paul say about childish thoughts in 1 Corinthians 13:11?

➢ Read 2 Corinthians 10:5. What did Paul say to do with thoughts that run contrary to God's Word?

Start keeping a list of the negative voices that tell you God will not deliver you. Devote a special place in your spiritual journal for this undertaking. Next to each negative voice, write what God has to say on the subject. Begin to memorize these Scripture affirmations so that when Satan brings doubt and fear, you will have a ready answer. There is no other way to bring your thoughts captive to the Word of God. Until you bring your negative thoughts captive to Christ, you will continue to cling to idols. Begin this work today.

Father, I know I fight an unseen enemy who wages war in the recesses of my mind. Help me bring every thought captive to the truth of Your Word [see 2 Corinthians 10:5].

O Lord, I will trust in You with all my heart and not rely on my understanding. I will acknowledge You in all my ways, confident that You will make my paths straight [see Proverbs 3:5-6].

DAY 4: *Our False Boundaries*

Because God has given us boundaries in all four areas of our lives, we have learned to construct false boundaries in the physical, mental, emotional and spiritual aspects of our being too. Physical false boundaries are usually easiest to spot. When we erect food as a false boundary, our shame becomes obvious to those around us, just as the crumbled walls of Jerusalem were a source of visible disgrace to the Jews.

Recall your answer to the question, "How do you usually react when you receive bad news?" on Day 2 of week two (page 26). The boxes you checked may point to false boundaries you have built. Most of us in First Place checked the box next to "Eat." We have learned to rely on food as a source of comfort, security and solace. We have also used food, and the resulting layer of body fat we accumulate, as a barrier of protection. Until we build healthy boundaries, our bodies will not let go of the weight we cling to for protection.

➤ What do you fear might happen if you reached and maintained your First Place goal weight?

➤ How do you think a smaller body would make you more vulnerable?

➤ What other physical barriers have you built for protection rather than relying on God to be your shield?

❑ Accomplishments   ❑ Money and possessions
❑ Busyness   ❑ Other people
❑ Clutter and disorganization ❑ Position and prestige
❑ Imagined illnesses   ❑ Other:

⋙ Jeremiah 9:23-24 tells us the real source of our security. What is to be our boast?

Is your relationship with the true and living God your source of significance? Explain your answer.

Before we can build healthy boundaries, we must identify and destroy all our false gods. Jesus was very clear with His disciples: We cannot serve two masters (see Matthew 6:24).

⋙ Read Joshua 24:14-16. Explain what Joshua said to the people regarding false boundaries. Conclude your writing with a declaration of whom you will serve.

 O Lord, You are my strength and my shield. My heart trusts in You and I am helped. You fill my heart with joy and cause my mouth to sing praises to You [see Psalm 28:7].

You are the Lord, my God, who takes hold of my hand and tells me not to fear, for You will help me [see Isaiah 41:13].

DAY 5: *Our Illusions*

Some of our false boundaries lay in the emotional and mental realm. Anger, guilt, depression, self-pity, complaining and feeling overwhelmed are just a few examples of the emotional barriers we put up rather than being transparent before God and crying out for His help.

➤ Look again at your answers to the question concerning how you handle bad news (page 26). Do any of your reactions reveal emotional or mental false boundaries?

God wants us to protect ourselves with His armor, not false boundaries of our own imagining. Ephesians 6:10-18 describes our God-given armor.

➤ According to this passage, what has God provided for our protection?

When we put on our God-given armor instead of turning to false boundaries, whose mighty power protects us (vv. 10-11)?

Satan knows he cannot prevail when we are shielded by divine protection, so he encourages us to rely on emotional and mental boundaries that resemble God-given emotions. Guilt is one such illusive, false emotional boundary. Many Christians fall into the trap of allowing accumulated guilt to keep them from crying out to God and asking for His help.

Second Corinthians 7:10 describes the difference between Godly sorrow and worldly sorrow.

Godly sorrow brings_____that leads to_____
and leaves no_____.
Worldly sorrow brings_____.

➤ According to Psalm 32:1-5, what does God do with our guilt when we confess our sins and turn to Him in repentance?

In his prophecy about the suffering servant, Jesus Christ, Isaiah vividly described the price that was paid for our sins. Read Isaiah 53. Now write a prayer thanking Jesus for coming to be a guilt offering so that you can experience the peace of God.

❧ In essence, what are you saying if you cling to guilt after you have confessed your sins to God? Let Paul's words in Galatians 5:1 help formulate your answer.

Does your answer coincide with the truth of God's Word? Remember, godly sorrow leaves no regret!

 Merciful God, I am blessed because my transgressions are forgiven and my sins are covered by the precious blood of Jesus, my Lord and Savior [see Psalm 32:1].
Precious Lord, forgive me when I devalue Your work on Calvary by clinging to my guilt and shame. By Your atoning sacrifice, You paid the price to set me free from guilt and to cleanse me from all unrighteousness. I accept Your precious gift of forgiveness with a grateful heart.

DAY 6: *Reflections*

This week we have looked at the false boundaries we have built rather than trusting solely in God and embracing the boundaries He has provided for our safety and protection. As our memory verse reminds us, God Himself is a shield around us, and He lifts up our heads from guilt and shame.

Some of the concepts we explored this week may be foreign to you. You may even feel confused or overwhelmed. Completing the Wellness Worksheets in the back of the book will help clarify the topics we've covered. As you ask God for wisdom and insight, He will send His gracious Spirit to guide you into all truth. You will begin to notice how you rely on other things—especially food—rather than crying out to God for help and allowing Him to be your rock and refuge.

Perhaps the false boundary of guilt threatens to keep you from acknowledging the truth. Feeling guilt can be much easier than feeling the pain and anxiety that comes with committing to the tough work of rebuilding our crumbled boundaries. Most of us don't change until the pain of not changing becomes greater than the pain of changing, and guilt keeps us from heeding pain's message.

One reason many of us struggle to lose weight is because we have not taken the time to rebuild our crumbled boundaries. As children, when we were powerless to stop those who violated our personal space, we learned to turn to food for comfort and protection. Perhaps food became synonymous with the love you craved as you grew up in a less-than-nurturing home. Perhaps you were abused verbally and emotionally, or even physically and sexually. Sadly, you may have often repeated those destructive relationship patterns in adulthood. Rather than doing the hard work of rebuilding your internal boundaries, have you compensated by erecting false boundaries that only lead to further abuse?

As you close today, determine to stop using food as a false boundary and ask God to empower you to rebuild your inner protection system. Yes, it is scary, but God is always part of the rebuilding process, and First Place is a safe environment in which to begin the work. Remember, God promises to be a shield around you, your rock and your refuge when you put your trust in Him.

Gracious God, You are the holy One who teaches me what is best and directs me in the way I should go [see Isaiah 48:17]. I will put my trust in You.

Lord, I am blessed when I believe that all You have said to me will be accomplished [see Luke 1:45].

O Lord, if You kept a record of sins, no one could stand [see Psalm 130:3]. Thank You for wiping my sins away like the morning mist [see Isaiah 44:22].

DAY 7: *Reflections*

When the Great Wall of China was built, Chinese leaders thought it was impregnable. It was fortified and well guarded. It seemed impossible that an enemy force could go over, under, around or through its expansive boundaries. The Chinese people felt safe from attack. However, the enemy easily breached the impressive barrier. Those who wanted to infiltrate China did not wage an open battle, nor did they try to scale the wall or attack the soldiers standing guard. None of that was necessary. All they had to do was bribe a gatekeeper.

God has given us a great wall of faith. It is our barrier—our shield of protection. As long as we humble ourselves under God's mighty hand and acknowledge Him as our shield and defender, we are kept safe by the strength of His power. Knowing this, Satan doesn't attack us head-on. Instead, like the enemy that wanted to invade China, the evil one tries to bribe the gatekeeper. Unable to attack us head-on, he works to infiltrate our hearts in small, seemingly harmless ways.

The devil's first tactic is to convince us there is no help for us in God. After that, he quickly presents us with the world's alternatives—things that bring temporary relief but ultimately lead to our demise. Then, once he has a toehold, our archenemy quickly establishes a stronghold. Those seemingly benign false boundaries that we refuse to let go of are the building blocks of the huge fortresses Satan uses to keep us from experiencing God's love. Satan seizes every opportunity to reinforce our faulty belief that God will not come to our defense. Nothing can keep us from enjoying an intimate relationship with our Father in heaven—*except* our stubborn refusal to bring those negative voices captive to the Word of

God. When we remain faithful to read and memorize Scripture and to pray continually, we bolster our defenses and guard our hearts against attack.

When we hide God's Word in our hearts, the enemy can't bribe the gatekeeper. We must always be on the alert and watch for the subtle ways in which the evil one tries to bribe us to gain entrance into our hearts, God's sacred dwelling place.

 Lord, I will hide Your Word in my heart so I will not fall victim to Satan's lies [see Psalm 119:11].

I love You, Lord, for You heard my voice; You heard my cry for mercy [see Psalm 116:1].

Some trust in chariots and some trust in horses, but I trust in Your name, O Lord, God of hosts [see Psalm 20:7].

NAME	REQUEST	RESULTS

HONOR GOD'S BOUNDARIES

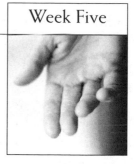

MEMORY VERSE

Humble yourselves, therefore, under God's mighty hand, that he may lift you up in due time.
1 Peter 5:6

If your personal boundaries have been shattered by heavy-handed authority figures, the thought of humbling yourself under God's mighty hand might be terrifying. You may have trouble separating humility—admitting we are finite human beings in need of God's help—from memories of painful humiliation, as others used their position of power to feed their egos at your expense. Yet if we expect God's blessing on our rebuilding efforts, we must build our boundaries within God's boundaries.

We cannot build our boundaries outside of God's righteous laws and decrees and expect Him to bless our efforts. God is a perfect parent who does not reward unacceptable behavior! Unless the Lord builds the house, its builders labor in vain (see Psalm 127:1). Before we begin to lay brick upon brick, we must be sure we are building according to God's plan, purpose and design for holy living. This week we will focus on the God who brings order out of chaos and invites us to humble ourselves under His mighty hand so that He can lift us up in victory.

DAY 1: *Order Comes from God*

The word "triage" usually describes a system of assigning priorities to medical treatment based on urgency, chance for survival and available resources—a system of establishing the order in which acts of assistance will be given. Whether for a personal heath crisis or a large-scale national emergency, a triage team is called in to establish a plan detailing what needs to be done immediately to save lives and restore well-being as efficiently as possible.

While we can all see the value of a triage center in a national disaster or life-threatening emergency, few of us realize the importance of making sure our daily activities are in sync with God's rhythm and design. As a result, we do not keep step with the Spirit. We allow less important things, sometimes even counterproductive things, to keep us from taking care of our top priorities.

The apostle Paul told the believers in Corinth that everything should be done "in a fitting and orderly way" (1 Corinthians 14:40). Those words echo the pattern we see throughout Scripture. God is a God of order, not of chaos and confusion. From the beginning, His plans have included an order in which things were accomplished.

➤ Read the creation account in Genesis 1:1-31, and then number the items below (1 to 7) to indicate when they were called forth.

_____Dry land and seas

_____Fish and birds

_____Humankind

_____Land animals

_____Light and darkness

_____Sun and moon

_____Vegetation

God created light before He created vegetation, which needs photosynthesis for growth. He created land and sea before He created fish and animals, which need water and dry ground for survival. He created food before He created living things, and the garden before He created the garden tenders. God made sure that everything was already in place to support each emerging part of His marvelous creation.

➤ How can you apply this principle of first things first to your involvement with First Place?

Our first priority is to seek God's kingdom and a right relationship with Him (see Matthew 6:33). Everything else will be added to us in proper order if we listen to God's voice and keep step with His Spirit.

I wait in hope for You, Lord; You are my hope and my shield [see Psalm 33:20].

Lord God, when I consider Your heavens, the work of Your hands and the moon and stars You have set in place, I am humbled to think that You are also mindful of me [see Psalm 8:3-4].

DAY 2: *Humility Comes Before Honor*

Our memory verse this week tells us another important truth about God's prescribed order: Humility precedes honor.

➤ Compare Peter's words about humility in 1 Peter 5:6 with Jesus' words in Matthew 23:12. What did you discover?

➤ Now turn to Psalm 139:5-6. What does David's song of praise reveal about humbling ourselves under God's mighty hand?

Part of God's design for each of us is to be hemmed in behind and before—to have boundaries that govern our activities. Part of humbling ourselves under His mighty hand is admitting that He is God and, as our creator, He knows what is best for us. When we purposefully go outside His boundaries and leave the protection of His almighty hand, we cannot expect His blessing.

Through the prophet Jeremiah, God told His wayward children that their rebellion had deprived them of good. Read Jeremiah 5:22-25 to see the connection between staying within God's boundaries and receiving His blessing.

≫ Paraphrase Jeremiah 5:22-25 to make it applicable to the First Place program.

Psalm 16:5-6 tells us another powerful truth about God's boundary lines.

≫ Who assigns your portion?

What does this allotted portion do?

≫ Where do God's boundary lines fall?

God's pleasant boundary lines include the Nine Commitments of First Place, which are in harmony with God's design and plan for His children. When we follow the First Place Live-It plan, we allow God to assign our portion and our cup and make our lives secure.

≫ Have you found that humility precedes honor in your First Place participation? Explain.

Until we are willing to let God determine our portions and willingly stay within His boundaries, we will not experience success in our First Place efforts.

≫ In what ways have you stepped outside God's boundary lines and yet expect to be rewarded for unacceptable behavior?

≫ What can you do today to bring your life into harmony with God's design and place yourself back within the boundary lines God has established for your good and His glory?

Gracious God, You are the strength of my heart and my portion forever [see Psalm 73:26].
You, O Lord, keep my lamp burning, You turn my darkness into light [see Psalm 18:28].

DAY 3: *Praise Comes Before Victory*

In our topsy-turvy, cart-before-the-horse society, we think of praise as something we do after the battle has been won or when the project is complete. We praise God in retrospect. However, God's Word tells us that we need to sing God's praises as a prelude to success.

Recall our study of Nehemiah's prayer during week two (Nehemiah 1:5-11). When confronted with bad news, the first thing Nehemiah did was pray.

≫ What was the first element of Nehemiah's prayer to God?

Nehemiah later praised God in response to the jeers of his opponents (see Nehemiah 2:20). Nehemiah used the weapon of praise over and over again as he led God's people to victory.

Nehemiah is not an isolated example of praise before victory. Scripture is full of examples of men and women who praised God before the battle and marched under the banner of God's protective right hand.

➤ What important truth does David state about praise in Psalm 8:2?

At the end of week two, we were introduced to Jehoshaphat. Let's return to that story to see how Jehoshaphat used praise as part of his battle tactic too. You might want to reread 2 Chronicles 20 to refresh your memory.

➤ According to 2 Chronicles 20:21, what happened after Jehoshaphat consulted with the people?

What did the appointed singers say?

The singers' praise reflected their trust in God to deliver them from their enemies. God was faithful to His word: Israel's enemies attacked and killed each other, eliminating the threat to Jehosaphat and his soldiers.

➤ What do you think might happen if you marched into your day-to-day battle against the forces of evil singing praise to God?

⟫ How can you specifically incorporate praise before victory into the First Place program?

Conclude today's lesson by singing a praise song or reciting a psalm of praise before you march into the busyness of your day. As you may have already noticed, many of the Scripture prayers in this Bible study are based on psalms of praise.

I will sing of your love and justice; to you, O Lord, I will sing praise [Psalm 101:1].
Great and marvelous are your deeds, Lord God Almighty. Just and true are your ways, King of the ages [Revelation 15:3].

DAY 4: *Confident Hope Comes from Obedience*

The apostle John gave us another foundational concept we must utilize as we begin to rebuild our boundaries within God's boundaries: Confident hope comes from obedience. Read 1 John 3:21-22 and complete the sentences below.

Dear friends, if our hearts do not_____us, we have before God and_____from Him anything we ask, because we_____His commands and do what_____Him.

⟫ What happens when your heart knows you are not obedient to God's commands (v. 21)?

What does that do to your confident hope in God's promises of provision and protection?

≫ How can you have confidence before God (v. 22)?

≫ John also tells us there is someone else who uses our disobedience to erode our confidence. What does Revelation 12:9-10 tell us about the accuser?

≫ According to Psalm 81:13-14, how can we subdue the voices of our foes?

≫ According to this week's memory verse, who are the ones God leads to victory?

≫ How is obedience part of humility?

As important as praise is to victory, we cannot separate praise from obedience. No matter what our lips say, we prove our love for God by joyfully obeying His commands. Humility acknowledges that we are finite human beings who need to continually yield our self-will to the sovereign will of God by respecting His boundaries.

Speaking through the prophet Isaiah, God warned His people about the folly of praising Him with their lips when their lives did not reflect their words.

➤ Summarize Isaiah 29:13 in your own words.

➤ Does the way you care for your body confess of the lordship of Christ? Explain.

➤ How does the way you care for your body affect your confidence before God?

➤ How can you make certain you have confidence before God and are not praising Him with your lips while your heart is far from Him?

Joyfully obeying the Nine Commitments of First Place also gives us confident hope because we know we are doing what pleases God.

O Lord, may Your hand be ready to help me, for I have chosen Your guidelines for life and happiness [see Psalm 119:173].
Almighty God, I rejoice in obeying You as one rejoices at finding great treasure (see Psalm 119:14).

DAY 5: *Commitment Has a Cost*

While grace is a free gift of God, commitment has a cost. In order for God's kingdom to be established in our hearts, our own little kingdoms must be surrendered to Him. We cannot serve two masters, and each day we must decide who is going to rule our lives. Jesus never minced words about the cost of discipleship. He challenged those who talked about making a commitment to Him to first consider the cost.

>> Carefully read Luke 14:25-33. What is the first cost Jesus told his disciples they would need to consider?

Verse 26 can be confusing. Remember, we must always interpret Scripture in the light of Scripture. Nowhere else does the Bible say we must hate our father and mother, spouse, children or siblings! Jesus was telling the crowd that compared to how much they were to love Him, it would be as if they hated everyone else. His point was that our relationship with Jesus must come before any earthly relationship.

>> Read Matthew 22:37. Write this greatest commandment in your own words.

>> What might rebuilding your crumbled boundaries cost you in terms of friendships and family relationships?

Is this a cost you are willing to pay?

The cost of losing friendships and relationships is steep, but the next thing Jesus told His would-be disciples they would have to give up is even more difficult.

➤ Reread Luke 14:26-27. What does following Jesus cost in terms of being in control of our lives?

What might this rebuilding project cost you in terms of priorities and plans?

Jesus gave the example of someone who wanted to build a tower. If the person did not consider the cost before the project was begun, he or she could run out of funds before the project was finished (see Luke 14:28-30).

➤ What did Jesus say would happen to the careless builder (vv. 29-30)?

➤ Rebuilding crumbled inner walls will take time and energy—and money. What are some of the resource costs you need to consider before you start to lay brick upon brick?

➤ Jesus also used the example of a king who was about to wage war. What did the king need to consider (vv. 31-32)?

The cost of discipleship can include resources of any kind: money, relationships, business affiliations, power, prestige, possessions, etc. Being willing to pay the cost is part of being a disciple.

Take a moment to consider the cost. Ask yourself if you are willing to begin this rebuilding project and see it through to completion. Write a prayer expressing both your commitment level and your concerns. If you commit to doing the work, leave the results to God.

 Precious Savior, You willingly paid the price of my redemption when You died so that I can have eternal life. I have carefully considered the cost of discipleship and have decided to follow You and willingly allow You to be the Lord of my life.

DAY 6: *Reflections*

At the beginning of his second letter, Peter gave another important principle we can apply as we rebuild our boundaries within God's boundaries: We aim for progress, not perfection.

> For this very reason, make every effort to add to your faith goodness; and to goodness, knowledge; and to knowledge, self-control; and to self-control, perseverance; and to perseverance, godliness; and to godliness, brotherly kindness; and to brotherly kindness, love. For if you possess these qualities in increasing measure, they will keep you from being ineffective and unproductive in your knowledge of our Lord Jesus Christ. But if anyone does not have them, he is nearsighted and blind, and has forgotten that he has been cleansed from his past sins (2 Peter 1:5-9).

We should strive to incorporate these qualities into our lives so that we can grow in Christian maturity; however, Peter does not say we are to attain these virtues all at once. Peter stressed the need to add them one at a time, in increasing measure, much the same way we would build a wall by placing one brick on top of the others until the project was complete.

Even Jesus—perfection embodied—"*grew* in wisdom and stature, and in favor with God and men" (Luke 2:52, emphasis added).

This week we have learned five important principles to incorporate into our boundary-rebuilding blueprint. Briefly review and list each of the five concepts.

Day 1—

Day 2—

Day 3—

Day 4—

Day 5—

Like the list in Peter's letter, these concepts are building blocks we must add one at a time and in increasing measure.

Place a check mark next to the principles you have already incorporated into your First Place regimen. Now use the principle of triage. Which of the items on the list do you need to add to your life first? Number the unchecked items by order of importance.

When we humble ourselves under the mighty hand of God, and bring our priorities in line with His, He will go before us as we rebuild our lives according to His plan and purpose.

Sovereign Lord, help me to obey Your commands so that my heart will not condemn me when I come to You in prayer [see 1 John 3:21-22].

Creator God, You looked at Your creation and declared it was good. Help me to care for my body in a way that brings You glory and honor [see Genesis 1:31].

Today I will humble myself under Your mighty hand so that You may lift me up in Your way and in Your time [see 1 Peter 5:6].

DAY 7: *Reflections*

It has been said that if Christians spent as much time praising God as they spend grumbling and complaining, they would soon have nothing to complain about! But even though our heads know the importance of praise and worship, our hearts have difficulty praising God. We are products of a not-enough society: discontent with what we have and always striving for more. Praise does not naturally roll off our lips. Yet God never asks us to do anything without first giving us all we need to respond obediently to His command. Right in the middle of your Bible is a marvelous book of praise songs suited to any and every occasion!

Psalms were the foundation of Jesus' prayer life. In the midst of incredible suffering, when His human capacity for thought and speech had been drained from His body, Jesus reverted to this default language as He prayed the words of Psalms. By hiding these precious praise verses in your heart, you too can always praise God, no matter what your circumstances. We can be sure the Lord of hosts is with us, working to confound our enemies, when our lips are singing His praises and our joyful obedience reflects the words that come from our mouths.

Spend some time today reading various psalms and adopt some of these time-tested praise songs as your own joyful songs before the Lord. Place the words on index cards and commit them to memory. Listed below are three praise verses to begin your collection. But don't stop here. Build on your personal Psalter verse upon verse until your heart and mind are overflowing with praise, no matter what the occasion.

Praise the Lord, O my soul. I will praise the Lord all my life; I will sing praise to my God as long as I live [Psalm 146:1-2].
Praise the Lord. How good it is to sing praises to our God, how pleasant and fitting to praise him! [Psalm 147:1].
Praise the Lord. Sing to the Lord a new song, his praise in the assembly of the saints [Psalm 149:1].

GROUP PRAYER REQUESTS   TODAY'S DATE:_____

NAME	REQUEST	RESULTS

TAKE ACTION THROUGH PRAYER

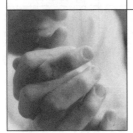

MEMORY VERSE
Devote yourselves to prayer,
being watchful and thankful.
Colossians 4:2

When faced with disturbing news, Nehemiah's heartfelt prayer allowed him to come up with an action plan. When King Artaxerxes asked Nehemiah how long the work would take and what supplies he needed to accomplish the task at hand, Nehemiah had a ready answer because he had already mentally planned his work through the process of prayer (see Nehemiah 1:4-5).

As we continue to look at the rebuilding of the wall, we will see that true prayer leads to action and action leads back to prayer. When we think of prayer as a means to an end, we miss the essence of our conversations with God. We become so focused on the outcome of our prayers that we fail to see them as part of the rhythm of our lives. This week we will learn how to be still and listen for God's voice as we learn to balance prayer and action, action and prayer.

In preparation for this week's study, read Nehemiah 4. Take special note of how action and prayer were combined as the workers did the tedious work necessary to rebuild the wall.

DAY 1: *Pray Hard*

We cannot rebuild healthy boundaries in isolation. The work is tedious and meticulous, often completed in the midst of hostile opposition. Without God's help, and the help of others, we are doomed to fail.

➣ Turn to 1 Thessalonians 5:16-18 to discover God's will for your life. Write these three short verses in the following space.

Read Ephesians 6:10-18. According to verse 18, when and how are we to pray?

Often we treat prayer as a mindless activity, but the apostle Peter went so far as to say that without an alert mind we cannot pray.

Read 1 Peter 4.7, and then write a short paragraph describing the correlation among alertness, prayer and self-control.

Peter learned that lesson firsthand. Read Matthew 26:40-41 and reflect on what Jesus said about watchfulness (alertness) and prayer. What did you discover?

Let's go back to Jerusalem and the wall-rebuilding efforts. In Nehemiah 4, the builders were tested by fierce opposition from their foes.

What were their enemies doing (vv. 1,8,11)?

In response to his enemies' anger, Nehemiah prayed, posted a guard day and night and continued rebuilding. We cannot post a physical guard day and night as we go about our work, yet we are far from defenseless.

Turn to Psalm 121. In what ways does God protect us?

Write a prayer of thanksgiving to the God who watches over you day and night.

Lord God Almighty, help me to be clear-minded and self-controlled so that I can pray words that are pleasing to Your ears [see 1 Peter 4:7].

O Lord, I can lie down and sleep in peace; I wake again because You sustain me [see Psalm 3:5].

DAY 2: *Develop the Right Attitude*

True prayer is not a babble of endless words attempting to convince God to do things our way. Heartfelt prayer is about our heart attitude, which is even more important than the words we pray.

➤ Turn to Matthew 6:5-8. What did Jesus say is more important than endless words?

Last week we learned some important concepts about order, humility, praise, obedience and commitment. In the space provided, write the words of the prayer Jesus gave His disciples in Matthew 6:9-13. Next to each sentence, explain how an attitude of order, humility, praise, obedience or commitment characterizes that part of the prayer. Some verses may contain more than one heart attitude. An example has been provided.

Verse	Attitude(s)
Our Father in heaven	*Humility—God is in heaven, I am not!*
	Praise—We can call God "Father;" He is approachable.

Perhaps the hardest concept to readily see is order, but look closely. Do you see the footprints of the God of order in the way the words of the prayer progress? Notice how each thought builds on the others.

➤ Reread Nehemiah 4:6. What were the workers' heart attitudes as they rebuilt the wall?

What was the result of their commitment to the work?

We need to bring a commitment to work with all ours hearts to our First Place boundary-rebuilding projects.

≫ Give concrete examples of how you are working with all your heart as you apply the Nine Commitments of First Place to your daily life.

≫ Drawing from last week's lesson on obedience, how does keeping the Nine Commitments of First Place on a consistent basis increase your confidence level that your Father in heaven will supply all your needs?

Close your quiet time today by mindfully praying the Lord's Prayer (Matthew 6:9-13). After you have concluded the prayer, write any new insights you have gleaned from those words in your prayer journal.

 Our Father in heaven, hallowed be Your name. Your kingdom come. Your will be done on earth as it is in heaven. Give us this day our daily bread. And forgive us our debts, as we forgive our debtors. And do not lead us into temptation, but deliver us from the evil one. For Yours is the kingdom and the power and the glory forever. Amen (Matthew 6:9-13, *NKJV*).

DAY 3: *Join the Ranks*

Yesterday we looked at the importance of having a right attitude when we pray—an attitude of humility, praise, obedience and commitment. We also looked at the words of the prayer Jesus taught His disciples in response to their request that He teach them to pray (see Matthew 6:9-13).

≫ What is the very first word of Jesus' prayer?

What other words do you find in these verses to indicate it is a corporate prayer? List the words and the verses in which you find them.

Earlier in the same passage Jesus told His disciples, "When you pray, go into your room, close the door and pray to your Father, who is unseen. Then your Father, who sees what is done in secret, will reward you" (Matthew 6:6).

➤ Since Scripture never contradicts Scripture, what do you think Jesus was teaching His disciples about prayer by giving these two examples?

➤ Reread Nehemiah 4:4,9,14 and 20. What do Nehemiah's words tell you about the nature of his prayers?

Nehemiah did not just pray for himself, he prayed for all those who were part of the rebuilding effort. As you rebuild your inner boundary walls, other members of your First Place group will be doing likewise. Although you cannot do their work for them, and they are not responsible for doing your work, prayer will bind your efforts.

Part of your First Place commitment is to pray for other group members. We are also to encourage one another with words that sustain us during our laborious work.

Look again at Nehemiah 4:14. Using this verse as a model, write on a piece of stationery a note of encouragement to your First Place prayer partner. Be sure to include words of order, praise, humility and hope that come from obedience and commitment regardless of the cost of rebuilding. End your note with a prayer invoking God's presence. If you cannot think of suitable words to invite God's blessing on his or her life, the priestly blessing of Numbers 6:24-26 is always appropriate!

Our Father, thank You for blessing me with fellow workers and comrades on this journey. I ask You to bless and keep them. Make Your face shine upon them and be gracious to them. Turn Your face toward them and give them peace (see Numbers 6:24-26).

DAY 4: *Work Double Duty*

No matter what our earthly occupations are, we each have a God-given vocation that is our most important work.

Read 2 Timothy 2:15 to learn about your primary vocation as a follower of Jesus.

➤ What does it mean to be a worker approved by God who does not need to be ashamed of his or her work?

➤ On a scale of 1 to 10, where would you rate your ability to correctly handle the Word of truth?

1	2	3	4	5	6	7	8	9	10
Apprentice							Master Artisan		

Why did you give yourself that rating?

➤ What can you do to become a worker approved by God, unashamed of your ability to properly handle His Word?

The builders working to restore the Jerusalem wall also had dual occupations. Nehemiah 4:16-18 gives us a description of their working conditions. According to verse 18, each builder wore a sword, ready to defend his work.

Of course, we aren't called to wear a real sword at our side as we go about our day; but there *is* a weapon we should always have close by. Read Ephesians 6:17 to discover this essential weapon.

Take the helmet of salvation and the_____of the Spirit, which is the _____.

➺ Which three of the Nine Commitments train us to be proficient in the use of our spiritual swords?

Though not limited to the Word of God, what other commitment is closely related to handling God's truth?

When we pray the words of Scripture, we combine two of the most powerful weapons in our spiritual arsenal.

➺ What does your rating at the beginning of this lesson tell you about your diligence in following the commitments that ask you to read, study, memorize and pray God's Word? (Remember, this rating may be a positive affirmation of your diligence and desire to become an approved worker.)

✎ Write Colossians 4:2 from memory in the space below. Also write a few sentences explaining how being able to correctly handle the Word of God will help you rebuild your boundaries.

 Lord God Almighty, I reach out my hands for Your commandments, which I love, and I meditate on Your decrees [see Psalm 119:48].

O Lord, I will praise You with an honorable heart as I continue to learn Your righteous laws [see Psalm 119:7].

DAY 5: *Respond to the Trumpet*

Working conditions were so hazardous along the Jerusalem wall that Nehemiah stationed workers in sight of one another. As he traveled along the wall to oversee the progress and encourage the workers, Nehemiah also kept with him a man with a trumpet.

✎ According to Nehemiah 4:20, what was the purpose of the trumpet?

What would be a modern-day equivalent to Nehemiah's trumpet?

When we are in need of encouragement or support, we can pick up the telephone and call someone in our First Place group or support network. Perhaps your church has a prayer chain that will summon the prayer warriors quickly when you are in need of prayer support.

On a separate piece of paper, make of list of people you can call when you need help. List several people because not everyone on your list will be available at all times. Keep this list in a place where you can find it quickly when trouble strikes. You may want to program some of the numbers into your telephone's memory system.

» Carefully reread Nehemiah 4:20. Upon arriving at the scene of someone's distress (in person or over the phone), what should your first response be?

Often we rush into crisis situations so quickly that we forget we are not the ones called to rescue others from their distress.

When the Israelites were in crisis beside the Red Sea, they went into panic mode. Read about their reaction in Exodus 14:10-12.

» In your own words, what did the Israelites say to Moses?

» Now read verses 13-14. How did Moses respond to their cries and complaints?

Who did Moses say would do the fighting?

What were the Israelites to do?

Once the people heeded Moses' words, the Lord told them what to do next: They were to move on (see v. 15). But until they were still before the Lord, they could not hear His instructions. A quiet time of prayer precedes efficient action.

Early in our studies we looked at Jehoshaphat's dilemma. Go back to 2 Chronicles 20:13-17.

⇒ What happened to the people as they stood before the Lord in stillness and prayer?

As much as we want to swing into immediate action and come to the rescue of our brothers and sisters in crisis, the most effective thing we can do is sit with them in stillness and pray. From that quiet time we will then be able to hear the Lord's voice saying, "This is the way; walk in it" (Isaiah 30:21).

Prayer leads to action; action leads to prayer. It is the rhythm of the Christian life. We work with the sword of the Spirit at our side, and we pray continually. From this posture we can be confident that our God will fight for us! We have only to be still and wait for His command.

Father, I am so thankful that You are near to me whenever I pray to You [see Deuteronomy 4:7].

Lord God, help me to be still and know that You are God [see Psalm 46:10].

DAY 6: *Reflections*

Healthy spiritual boundaries allow us to determine where we stop and God begins. Some religions confuse the boundary between God and man by saying that "you are God" or "you are divine." However, Christianity is based on having a right relationship with God. We are to be *like* God in character, but we are not called to *be* God. No matter how mature we become in our Christian walk, we will always be finite human beings striving for relationship with the true and living God. Even in heaven we will not be one with God. We will be among the heavenly masses singing His praises throughout eternity. We may laugh at the thought of being God, but at times each of us tries to play God in our own life or in the lives of others.

Our spiritual boundaries are severely tested when those we care about suffer a crisis. Even Moses, God's faithful servant, did not enter the Promised Land because in a high-stress moment, his spiritual boundaries became blurred. The Israelites were thirsty. They were grumbling and complaining. God spoke to Moses, saying, "Take the staff, and you and your brother Aaron gather the assembly together. Speak to that rock before their eyes and it will pour out its water. You will bring water out of the rock for the community so they and their livestock can drink" (Numbers 20:8). But instead of speaking to the rock, Moses struck it twice with his staff shouting, "Listen, you rebels, must we bring you water out of this rock?" (v. 10). Water gushed out of the rock for the community, but the Lord said to Moses and Aaron, "Because you did not trust in me enough to honor me as holy in the sight of the Israelites, you will not bring this community into the land I give them" (Numbers 20:12). How did Moses not honor God as holy? He forgot who he was and said, "must *we* bring you water," as if it were in his power to save the people (v. 10, emphasis added). Instead of speaking to the rock, Moses struck it in an attempt to show his might and his power rather than giving glory to God.

Like Moses, we often forget who we are. We rush into crisis situations and try to solve problems in our own strength and power. We want to rescue those in distress from their misery and pain. In the process, we may interrupt the very test God is using to teach those we attempt to rescue— a powerful lesson in trust and obedience.

We are not the Savior. Our job—our *only* job—is to point those in crisis to the One who can rescue them from distress. We are the messengers, not the Message. Psalm 146:3 exhorts us not to put our trust in mortal men, who cannot save. We are to put our trust in God, for only He can redeem us from the pit, forgive our sins, heal all our diseases and satisfy our desires (see Psalm 103:2-4).

Healthy spiritual boundaries tell us where we end and where God begins. They allow us to pray continually and be used as God's servants as He does His work of redeeming a lost and fallen world. Healthy spiritual boundaries allow us to be still and let God fight for us.

O Lord, I am blessed because You are my God [see Psalm 144:15].

Father, hear my prayer and listen to my cry for mercy; in Your faithfulness and righteousness rescue me [see Psalm 143:1].

You are my refuge and my strength. You are always ready to help me in times of crises [see Psalm 46:1].

DAY 7: *Reflections*

A young monk had questions about his order's motto, "pray and work." To him, the two words were contradictory. If he truly trusted in prayer, why did he need to continue to work? If he was going to work, why bother to pray? The abbey was located near the shore of a large lake and one day the abbot invited the confused novice to row across the lake with him. The abbot began to row but with only one oar in the water. As a result the boat went in circles, and they made no progress. The young monk said, "Abbot, unless you row with both oars, we won't get anywhere." The abbot replied, "You're so right, son! The right oar is prayer; the left is work. Unless you use them together, you'll just go in circles."

Prayer is not a passive activity. It requires asking, seeking and knocking. In the words of many a saint, it is a combination of working like there is no prayer and praying like there is no work. First Place teaches us to balance work and prayer. We know the balance is correct when we quit going in circles and begin walking in sync with the Spirit. Through prayer God gives us guidance and direction, and enables us to do the work that will allow our petitions to become reality. Work then sends us back to prayer as we realize we can only keep the Nine Commitments of First Place by spending quiet time abiding in God. Prayer and work comprise the rhythm that allows us to live balanced lives. We will quit going in circles when we have learned the secret of the motto "pray and work."

Almighty God, help me find the rhythm of prayer and work, work and prayer, so that I can walk in sync with Your Spirit.

Thank You, Father, that because of Christ I can approach You with confidence and receive mercy and help in my time of need [see Hebrews 4:16].

Sovereign Lord, help me to devote myself to prayer and to be watchful and thankful as I put my trust in Your unfailing love [see Colossians 4:2].

GROUP PRAYER REQUESTS   TODAY'S DATE:_____

NAME	REQUEST	RESULTS

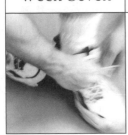
EXPECT OPPOSITION

MEMORY VERSE
*You were running a good race. Who cut in
on you and kept you from obeying the truth?*
Galatians 5:7

Commitment and opposition always go hand in hand. Throughout salvation history we see this pattern over and over. Whenever someone makes a commitment to serve God, the evil one always lurks in the shadows, ready to stomp that commitment into failure. The good news is that we can learn to anticipate this cycle and, knowing this truth, can prepare ourselves for what lies ahead. As soon as we make a commitment to spiritual growth and change, we can expect immense opposition in our everyday environments. We can expect to be bombarded from every direction by people, places and things that will test our resolve and dampen our desire to persevere. The evil one is always close at hand to fill our minds with doubt, deception and denial, and to tempt us with old, destructive habits.

This week we will look at the enemy's wiles, visible and invisible, that threaten to cut in on us and keep us from obeying the truth. Paul told the Corinthians to be aware of Satan's schemes so that the devil could not outwit them (see 2 Corinthians 2:11). Paul's words also ring true for believers today.

DAY 1: *Identify the Real Enemy*

Early in our study of Nehemiah's rebuilding project, we were introduced to evil forces that would oppose Nehemiah's efforts and threaten his plans. Go back to Nehemiah 2.

➤ Who were Nehemiah's visible enemies (vv. 10,19)?

Why were these enemies disturbed by Nehemiah's plans?

What was their first oppositional tactic (v. 19)?

It is easy to focus so much attention on the threats and jeers of the visible enemy that we fail to see who is behind the opposition. Revelation 12:9 calls Satan an "ancient serpent" who "leads the whole world astray." He is our archenemy, working behind the scenes to carry out his diabolical plans.

➤ Turn to Ephesians 6:12. What insight do Paul's words give us about the enemy against whom we struggle?

➤ Recall the story Jesus told about two fathers in John 8:42-44. Who were these two fathers?

How does Jesus describe the evil father's desire (v. 44)?

Jesus was very clear: We either belong to one father or the other. There is no neutral ground. Those who belong to God do the will of their Father in heaven. Those who belong to Satan are used as pawns to carry out his schemes. In writing to young Timothy, the apostle Paul called the devil's subjects captives.

≫ Read 2 Timothy 2:24-26, and then write verse 26 in your own words.

≫ Although the villains in the book of Nehemiah had names such as Sanballat, Tobiah and Geshem, who was the real enemy trying to sabotage Nehemiah's plans?

Our opponents may take many forms, but Satan is the controlling force behind those who attempt to thwart our plans and keep us from doing what pleases God.

Identifying the real enemy allows us to fight the spiritual battle with spiritual weapons. These weapons are described in Ephesians 6:10-18. Review the list carefully.

≫ Which weapon do you need to employ today in your struggle against evil?

How is the First Place program part of your arsenal against Satan's attacks?

Sovereign Lord, thank You for giving me divine weapons to fight against the spiritual forces that threaten my plans to do what is pleasing to You.

Abba Father, Jesus died so that I could be included in Your family and call You my Father. As a member of Your family, I will strive to do Your will, even in the face of opposition and temptation.

DAY 2: Brace Yourself for Attack

Because our primary struggles against the forces of evil are fought in the battleground of our minds, that is where Satan stages his initial attack. Our enemy knows that hostile words can undermine our confidence in God and erode our resolve to make positive change.

In week two we identified the voice of the enemy. Reread Psalm 3:1-2 to refresh your memory. Now turn to Nehemiah 4:2-3 and read what Sanballat and Tobiah had to say about the Jews. Verbal attack is often the enemy's next offensive maneuver.

➤ What was Nehemiah's first defense against their verbal attack (vv. 4-5)?

When faced with verbal assault, we often try to retaliate in kind. But notice that Nehemiah did not try to debate with his enemies. He did not try to verbally defend his position. He took his complaint directly to God.

➤ Read Psalm 55:16-19. Write a short description of how David handled his enemies' verbal attacks.

Recall from Genesis 3:1-5 that when Satan tempted Eve, she fell into his trap long before she took a bite of the forbidden fruit. Instead of going directly to God with her questions, Eve tried to answer the crafty serpent with her own words.

When faced with evil, we must learn not to dialogue, debate, dispute or dabble in polite conversation. When we take our complaints and questions to God, He will be our defender. All we need do is stand firm in His mighty power and let Him deal with our attackers' hostile words.

➤ In what area(s) of your life are you trying to dispute, dialogue, debate or dabble in conversation with the enemy?

➤ Review Matthew 4:1-11. When Jesus was under verbal attack, how did He respond?

How can you use your Scripture memory commitment in your struggle against evil?

➤ What have you learned from today's lesson that will help you stop the enemy's first tactic as he tries to thwart your plans and keep you from obeying the truth?

 Gracious Lord, thank You for giving me Your Word so that I will not be thrown off track by the devil's schemes.

Lord, when I am in doubt and don't know what to do, I will take my fears to You in prayer and allow You to be my strong defender.

DAY 3: *Be Ready for Plan B*

When verbal attacks fail, the enemy does not retreat in failure. He simply resorts to plan B, and when plan B fails he tries plan C. Satan is relentless in trying to eradicate truth. Rather than admitting he has been defeated, our ancient enemy goes into hiding and waits for an opportune time to up the ante.

➤ Read Nehemiah 4:7-12. When hostile words did not stop the work on the wall, what did the opposition begin to do?

One of the devil's second-level strategies is physical violence. When ridicule did not stop Nehemiah's efforts, his opponents resorted to threats of physical harm. Sadly, this is not an isolated scriptural account of physical harm.

> Read John 11:45-53. Centuries after the book of Nehemiah was written, what did the Jewish leaders do when they could not verbally intimidate Jesus?

> In Matthew 2:1-17 we are introduced to another enemy of Christ. Read this familiar story and identify both the villain and his plot.

What did Joseph and Mary do to protect their child from their enemy's evil plan (vv. 13-15)?

When we begin to build healthy boundaries that keep us from being manipulated by those hungry for power and control, at times we too may be in physical danger. Turn to the list you made in week three, Day 5, of the people who may oppose your boundary-rebuilding efforts (page 47). Look over this list prayerfully. Is there anyone on this list that you fear might resort to physical violence when you begin to set limits and boundaries that threaten his or her position of power and control?

If so, like Joseph and Mary, you may also have to flee for safety until your abuser can be subdued. Domestic violence is a very real tragedy in today's society. Part of being response-able is having a plan in place to deal with those who pose a threat to your safety, or the safety of your children. Make an appointment to talk to your pastor or a trained counselor if you feel you are in danger. Take whatever steps necessary to protect yourself. Physical violence is never to be tolerated. Feeling sorry for the enemy or trying to justify his or her actions will not solve the problem. This is a time for swift and decisive action.

➤ Turn back to Nehemiah 4:14. What might God be calling you to do to help your brothers, sisters, sons and daughters who are being abused?

Close today's lesson in prayer for those who are victims of domestic violence.

 God of power and might, You tell me to speak up for those who cannot speak for themselves and to defend the rights of the needy [see Psalm 82:3-4].

Help me never to be in denial about domestic violence. Give me discernment and courage to flee if I am in danger and to always be willing to help others escape the danger of physical harm.

DAY 4: *Beware of Subtle Tactics*

Sometimes the enemy does not resort to physical violence. When verbal threats fail, the enemy often resorts to distraction as a way of keeping us from obeying the truth. Read Nehemiah 6:1-4 to gain insight into how this tactic works.

➤ What did Nehemiah's enemies do in a subtle attempt to distract him from his primary task?

How many times was the invitation sent (v. 4)?

What was Nehemiah's reply each time they asked him to stop his work to meet with them (v. 3)?

≫ What invitations might you need to turn down if you are going to concentrate your time, attention and effort on your boundary-rebuilding project?

Nehemiah had the discernment to recognize the invitation for what it really was: a distraction that would stop him from working and a threat to his life. Think back to what we have learned about Nehemiah in previous lessons.

≫ How do you think Nehemiah had the ability to discern the truth about the enemy's motives?

≫ What can you learn from Nehemiah's example about discerning whether to accept invitations that may interfere with what God has called you to do?

When his enemies could not distract Nehemiah, they tried two more subtle tactics in an attempt to thwart his plans (see Nehemiah 6:5-14). First, they made up lies in a vain attempt to stop the work. When a polite invitation failed to produce results, they tried to goad Nehemiah into defending his motives. Next, they tried to discredit Nehemiah so that the people would lose confidence in him. In his usual fashion, Nehemiah discerned their plots and took his complaint to God, asking God to repay his enemies for trying to stop the good work he was doing.

How can you begin to use your prayer time to discern the subtle ways the enemy may be attempting to keep you from obeying the truth?

Write this week's memory verse in the space below. After you have written the verse, compose a prayer asking God to give you wisdom and discernment so that you can determine those things that threaten to keep you from doing the good work God has called you to do.

Holy and loving God, so many things threaten to throw me off course and sabotage my desire to do what is pleasing to You. As soon as I begin rebuilding, things that I am powerless to control cut in on me.

Lord, You know my struggle and the desire of my heart. Help me to discern the motives and actions of others so that I can do what is pleasing to You and not be distracted by Satan's schemes.

DAY 5: *Put It All Together*

This week we have looked at a variety of tactics the enemy employs in his never-ending attempt to keep us from obeying the truth. Remember, we are not to be ignorant of the devil's schemes! Reflect on all the ways the enemy tried to stop Nehemiah's rebuilding project.

⇛ What ways might the enemy try to sabotage your plans? The devil's wiles are not limited to those in our study. Be creative as you think of the ways he might effectively cut you off as you endeavor to carry out God's plans.

⇛ Hebrews 12:1 gives us further insight into the ways Satan might attempt to stop us from persevering in our efforts. What sins has Satan used in the past to hinder and entangle you?

Do you think Satan knows what your weak points are? Certainly he does! That is why it is so important to be aware of the things that have worked for him in the past. Remember, our first line of defense is awareness. Go back over your list and be sure you have been honest about the sins that easily entangle you.

⇛ Look again at the list you just made. If you were the enemy, what would you do in the future to trip you up?

⇛ What can you do to shore up your weaknesses so that you will not be easy prey for the enemy's attack?

⇛ For most of us in the First Place program, our disordered relationship with food is a weak spot. How can the Nine Commitments of First Place strengthen this weakness and shore up your defenses?

Our memory verse asks us to examine our failures. Paul told the Galatians they had been running a good race, but then something cut in and threw them off track.

➣ What cuts in on you as you run the good race and strive to obey the truth?

Write a prayer thanking God for giving you awareness so that you can confess your sins, accept His forgiveness, put your past behind you and redouble your efforts as you work to live a life pleasing to Him.

My Lord and my God, You invite me to leave the past behind so that I can run the race You have set before me [see Philippians 3:13]. Today I accept Your gracious offer of forgiveness.

Sovereign Lord, the wiles of the enemy are subtle and deceptive, but You have given me Your Spirit to lead me into all truth. Thank You for promising You will never leave me to face my problems alone.

DAY 6: *Reflections*

When trying to eliminate sin from our lives, a critical strategy is to recognize our vulnerability, accept it and avoid situations and places that set us up for failure. To win the battle we must learn to cut off the enemy's supply routes. We must learn to starve sin. This may mean completely avoiding certain people, places and things because of the magnetic pull their influence exerts over us. Satan knows our weaknesses and uses all the tools at his command to keep us in spiritual jeopardy. If we are serious about eliminating sin from our lives, we must stop gravitating to places that allow us to gratify the desires of our sinful nature. If we find that certain situations continually undermine our resolve and contribute to drinking, overeating, impulse buying, gossiping or whatever else gratifies our sinful nature, then we must eliminate those situations if we are going to stand strong against the wiles of the evil one.

Although at times we feel like we are the ones on a diet, the real purpose of the First Place program is to starve sin. By putting Christ first in all things, there is no room for our sinful nature to thrive. If we are serious about the First Place program, we will quickly learn to identify those people, places and things that keep us from reaching our goals. Often what lures us away from our resolve is not food.

Look for consistent patterns in the ways Satan tempts you. Those are the people, places and circumstances you must eliminate. You are not on a diet—you are learning to give Christ first place in your life so you can starve sin by cutting off the enemy's supply routes. Take time today to identify the things that jeopardize your success in the First Place program so that you can cut off the supply routes. Write those things in the space provided.

Gracious God, I have hidden Your Word in my heart so that I won't sin against You [see Psalm 119:11].

Father, I know I cannot conquer the enemy by giving in to his wiles. Help me to resist the devil, confident that when I resist he will flee from me [see James 4:7].

O Lord, strengthen my hands so that I can complete the work You have put before me [see Nehemiah 6:9].

DAY 7: *Reflections*

The spiritual dimension of First Place is essential to success because of the opposition we face. Through the spiritual commitments of Bible study, Scripture reading, prayer and Scripture memory, we draw from a power inside us that is greater than the temptations that surround us. Most of us join First Place because we want to lose weight, but when we make the First Place program just about what we eat, we set ourselves up to fail. In addition to mental resolve, we need divine weapons to ward off the attacks of the evil one, who waits on the sidelines, ready to lure us into temptation and sabotage our plans. First Place is about balance and reliance on the strength of the Holy Spirit to overcome the strongholds that we are powerless to overcome on our own.

Whenever we make a commitment to serve God and do the work He has put before us, we need to be mindful of the commitment-temptation cycle (i.e., heightened temptation always follows renewed commitment). Awareness allows us to protect ourselves with the whole armor of God so that we can stand firm in His mighty power and resist the wiles of the evil one.

Review the lists you made on Day 5 (pages 107-108). Spend some time in prayer asking God to send His Spirit to reveal any other areas of weakness you have been in denial about. God does not want you to be ignorant about the devil's schemes. You honor God when you admit your weaknesses and ask Him to be your strength.

Our best defense is a strong offense. While being faithful to the First Place program, you will be able to hear God's voice and have confidence in prayer because of your obedience to Him. Remember, Satan's tactics are often subtle. He is a master of disguise and deception, and the father of lies. Arm yourself with awareness and put on the full armor of God so that you can stand firm in His might and power. Finally, be encouraged. Jesus told His disciples, "In this world you will have trouble. But take heart! I have overcome the world" (John 16:33). Those are His words to you too. When you arm yourself with His might and power, you will be victorious. He has won the battle! If God is for you, you cannot fail.

Thank You, Lord, for assuring me of victory because You have overcome the world [see John 16:33].

Father, You are great and awesome, and You will fight for me when I put my trust in You.

Give thanks to the Lord, for he is good. His love endures forever [Psalm 136:1].

GROUP PRAYER REQUESTS   TODAY'S DATE:_____

NAME	REQUEST	RESULTS

COMBAT FATIGUE AND FRUSTRATION

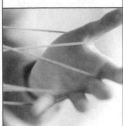

MEMORY VERSE
*Never be lacking in zeal, but keep your
spiritual fervor, serving the Lord.*
Romans 12:11

About halfway through the rebuilding of the wall, Nehemiah's workers fell prey to two other enemies: fatigue and frustration. Nehemiah 4:10 tells us the workers were tired and there was rubble everywhere. They were under constant threat of attack, and they worked from the first light of morning until the sun set each day (see v. 21). Their strength was giving out, their enthusiasm had waned, and they were only halfway done! Though their external enemies could not defeat the Israelites, an invisible enemy threatened to defeat them from within.

During the long, tedious job of rebuilding our boundaries, especially in the face of opposition, we also will experience fatigue and frustration from the stress of working under less-than-ideal circumstances day in and day out. At times we may feel buried under the rubble and debris as the Holy Spirit does His work in us. Though not yet functioning at full capacity, our workload will not diminish. We will need time to grieve our losses and to grapple with our new roles and identities. We will become weary and tired as change becomes the order of the day. Knowing these trials are ahead, we must pace ourselves for the long haul and prioritize, lest we lose heart and cave in to fatigue and frustration.

DAY 1: *Pace Yourself*

Rebuilding the crumbled walls and restoring the burned gates was neither quick nor easy. Turn to Nehemiah 6:15 and record how long the rebuilding project took.

So the wall was_____on the twenty-fifth of Elul,
in_____days.

It took Nehemiah and his band of workers almost two months to
complete their work. Remember, they did not have power equipment,
tractors or cement trucks. This was tedious, backbreaking work, from
sunup to sundown!

➤ Carefully reread Nehemiah 4 and summarize the working conditions
and hazards. Write as though you are giving a report to a labor review
board.

Not only were Nehemiah and his men doing heavy labor, but they
were also doing it in a war zone!

➤ Nehemiah 4:6-10 states when frustration and fatigue began to take its
toll. Where were the workers in the rebuilding process when their
enthusiasm began to wane (v. 10)?

As we have already learned, the Bible becomes real for us when we
begin to make the stories relevant to our own experiences. With this in
mind, compose an account of the conditions you have labored under since
beginning your First Place endeavors and where you are in relation to
your goal. Include pertinent details about extra stressors that have added
to your workload and whether your initial enthusiasm has given way to
discouragement and despair. Also tell about any hostile opposition or
insults you have endured as you have struggled to restore your body to
health and vitality. Once again, write your words as though you were
preparing a report for a labor review board.

Even though times were tough, Nehemiah continually praised the Lord for His faithfulness. Nehemiah encouraged the people to "Remember the Lord, who is great and awesome" (Nehemiah 4:14). Can you praise God for sustaining you thus far in your First Place journey? Write a short prayer of thanksgiving, praising God for His faithfulness and love.

 O Lord, I will give You thanks, for You are good and Your love endures forever [see Psalm 118:1].
Loving Father, Your mercies are fresh every morning. Great is Your faithfulness [see Lamentations 3:22-23].

DAY 2: *Keep a Balanced Perspective*

Look again at Nehemiah 4:6. We must be careful not to overlook one word that helps us understand the rebuilding process.

So we rebuilt the wall till_____of it reached half its height, for the people worked with_____their heart (Nehemiah 4:6).

Often we approach the First Place program as we approach a smorgasbord deli line. We take a double helping of the commitments that are easy for us to digest and pass up the things that are hard for us to chew and swallow! But until we devote ourselves to all the commitments with all our heart, we are not really participating in First Place! When we insist on doing it our way—the easy way—we deprive ourselves of the balance of this wonderful program. Like it or not, half measures do not produce complete results.

The Nine Commitments of First Place are listed below. Above each commitment are columns. Create a bar graph above each commitment indicating your level of participation.

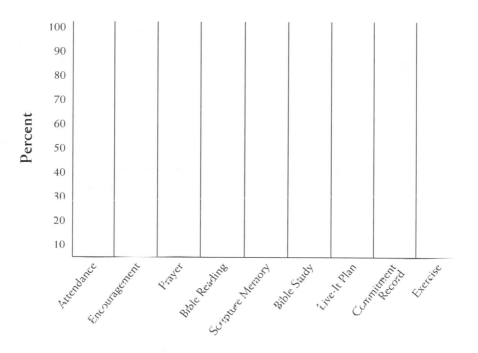

Nine Commitments

≫ If you have not given all Nine Commitments equal priority, explain the differentiation.

≫ What do you need to change so that you can say you have worked at *all* your First Place commitments with *all* your heart?

We see the word "all" in another important scriptural principle. Look up Matthew 22:37-38, and then describe the importance of this word.

Do your graph results show that you are taking this passage to heart? Explain.

Close today's session by writing a prayer of confession, asking God to renew your heart and mind and to give you wholehearted devotion in the weeks ahead.

 Almighty God, thank You for loving me, even when I do not love You with all my heart or care for my body as a reflection of my love for You.

Create in me a pure heart, O God, and renew a steadfast spirit within me [Psalm 51:10].

DAY 3: Come Away and Rest

Though the second greatest commandment is to love others as much as we love ourselves (see Matthew 22:39), we are not called to neglect caring for ourselves in the process. Being a self-made martyr who suffers from the fatigue of endless service is all too often thought of as a Christian virtue; however, Scripture shows us a different model.

⟩⟩ A stream of needy people continually bombarded Jesus and His disciples. In your Bibles, turn to Mark 6:30-31. What did Jesus say to His frazzled disciples?

Rest is a Christian virtue that we often dismiss in the busyness of our days. Yet rest is as much a part of God's created order as work!

⟩⟩ What does each of the following Scriptures teach us about rest?

Genesis 2:2

Exodus 31:15

Leviticus 25:5

Deuteronomy 33:12

Psalm 127:2

Proverbs 19:23

Matthew 11:28

Acts 6:1-4

≫ Refer back to the bar graph you created in yesterday's lesson. Does compulsive busyness keep you from participating in First Place whole-heartedly? Explain.

We often pray for God's blessing without realizing that one of His most precious and most easily attainable blessings is rest. Take some time today to rest between God's shoulders to prevent the fatigue and frustration of self-imposed busyness that, in the name of service, keeps you from honoring God with your body.

 Lord, thank You for knowing I am weary and for inviting me to come away with You and rest. Help me sit at Your feet and learn from You instead of being distracted by all the preparations to be made [see Luke 10:40-42].

Jesus, I am so thankful that Your burden is light [see Matthew 11:30]. Teach me to let go and to let You carry my heavy burdens for me.

DAY 4: *Savor Each Moment*

True rest is not just lack of physical activity; it is also freedom from anxiety and stress. We know all too well the physical health effects of unrelenting stress. Anxiety is a toxic poison that slowly kills our bodies, minds, hearts and spirits.

The intensity of the physical labor was not the only problem the Jerusalem wall builders struggled with. Living in a constant state of anxiety contributed greatly to their fatigue and frustration.

≫ Turn back to Nehemiah 4:11-12. What do these verses tell you about the workers' stress levels?

What were they afraid of?

Anxiety is fear projected into the future. At its root, anxiety is a lack of trust in God's providence, protection and ongoing provision.

➤ Read what Jesus told His disciples about worry in Matthew 6:25 and Matthew 10:19. Was Jesus addressing future or present needs? What key phrases support your answer?

What do these verses tell you about obsessing over future events?

➤ The apostle Paul also addressed the subject of anxiety in Philippians 4:6-7. According to these verses, what are we supposed to do with our projected needs?

➤ According to 1 Peter 5:7, what should we do with our anxiety?

Why don't we need to be worried about the future?

➤ Finally, turn to Luke 21:34. What two things did Jesus list with the "anxieties of life" that keep us from watching and praying?

Both items Jesus listed are forms of overindulgence. What insight about the nature of anxiety do His words give you?

➤ Write 1 Peter 5:7-8 in the space below.

After reading what Jesus had to say about the anxieties of life being akin to dissipation and drunkenness, why do you think Peter links anxiety with being self-controlled and alert?

➤ How much of your fatigue and frustration might be the result of an anxiety hangover?

➤ What have you learned from today's lesson about feelings of anxiety?

Write a short prayer casting your anxiety onto God and expressing your confidence in His loving care, both now and in the future.

Lord God, You are the same yesterday, today and forever [see Hebrews 13:8]. I will put my trust in Your provision and not give in to the self-indulgence of anxiety.

Merciful and loving God, I am confident You will supply all my needs according to Your glorious riches in Christ Jesus [see Philippians 4:19]. When I am tempted to give in to worry I will cast my cares on You [see 1 Peter 5:7].

DAY 5: Build Your "No" Muscle

Exercise is one of the Nine Commitments of First Place. Go back to Day 2 and see where you ranked exercise on your bar graph. For many of us, exercise is one of those things we somehow can't manage to make time for. In the busyness of our days, exercise is relegated to "Someday I'll." Yet exercise is an essential part of the fitness needed to endure the daily stress of life without giving in to fatigue and frustration.

Before proceeding with today's lesson, turn to pages 74 and 75 of your *First Place Member's Guide* and review the many benefits of physical exercise.

➤ In the space below write Romans 12:11 from memory.

➤ How are the benefits of physical exercise related to zeal, spiritual fervor and serving the Lord?

≫ Look up Acts 20:13-14. Why do you think Paul might have chosen to walk?

Traveling on foot not only provided physical exercise, but it also afforded Paul an opportunity to walk with the Lord in quiet conversation and to listen for the Spirit's voice giving him direction and discernment. Have you ever considered combining exercise and prayer?

≫ List at least two specific ways you can exercise your body and build your relationship with God at the same time.

Being physically fit is an important part of being zealous and serving the Lord with a joyful heart. Yet as important as physical exercise is to our well-being, there is another muscle we all need to exercise daily in order to serve the Lord with zeal and spiritual fervor: our "no" muscle. To succeed in First Place, we must develop boundaries that allow us to purposefully select what is important and selectively reject the things that distract us and keep us from obeying the truth. Rather than flitting from one activity to another, looking for instant gratification, we must focus on achieving our goals. This will mean exercising our "no" muscle so that we can say yes to the Nine Commitments of First Place. Our "no" muscle may be the flabbiest muscle we have! Yet without single-minded focus, things will continue to cut us off and keep us from doing the things that are important to God—things like caring for our body, mind, emotions and spirit.

Look again at your Day 2 bar graph. Could the reason you have not been able to devote all your heart to the Nine Commitments of First Place be because you have a flabby "no" muscle? Remember, in order to purpose-fully select what is important, we must purposefully reject the things that distract us and keep us in a state of frustration and fatigue.

≫ List five things you need to say no to so that you can say yes to the Nine Commitments of First Place on a consistent basis. Then begin exercising your "no" muscle today.

1.

2.

3.

4.

5.

Father, help me to say no to those things that keep me distracted, anxious and tired so that I can wholeheartedly say yes to You.

Lord God, I am fearfully and wonderfully made [see Psalm 139:14]. Help me to honor You by caring for my body as the temple of Your Holy Spirit.

DAY 6: *Reflections*

We all have those sluggish, gloomy, listless days when we just can't seem to do anything but sit around. Some call those days the doldrums, referring to the dull, low-spirited time that predictably follows a tantrum. After the flurry of frenzied activity that accompanies an adrenaline rush, our bodies, minds, emotions and spirits shut down. When we take an honest look at ourselves, most of us can point to a cycle of hyperactivity followed by a time of being in the doldrums. We go at a frantic pace for days and then crash, like pebbles skipping across a pond until they lose their momentum and plunge into the depths of the water.

There is actually a place located near the equator named the Doldrums, appropriately titled because of the shifting winds, calms and squalls in the area. A sailing ship caught in the Doldrums could be stranded for days due to lack of wind. In the midst of the doldrums, our lives come to a standstill too. We cease to care for our bodies, minds or spirits, whereas a diligent man or woman prizes his or her possessions and practices self-care. Pacing ourselves through self-disciplined activity that includes moderation and planned times of rest is a much healthier lifestyle than uncontrolled hyperactivity followed by the doldrums.

Both ends of the destructive cycle—hyperactivity and doldrums—are danger zones for those of us in First Place. When we are hyperactive, our eating is out of control and we are either "too busy" to exercise or we exercise in excess. Then we swing down to the doldrums, where we face the temptation to overeat in a vain attempt to raise our sagging spirits, and we are "too tired" to exercise. We can find balance and moderation within First Place by keeping the Nine Commitments daily and learning to keep in step with the Spirit. We cannot take care of ourselves as God commands as long as we stay caught in the up-and-down cycle of tantrums and doldrums.

Take time today to carefully examine your life. Do you see a pattern of hyperactivity followed by a bout of the doldrums? If so, protect your body, mind, emotions and spirit by diligently applying the balance and moderation of the First Place program to every area of your life.

Lord, "I have considered my ways and have turned my steps to your statutes" [Psalm 119:59].

Almighty God, help me exercise my body and my mind so that I can live a life that pleases You.

Gracious Father, today I will cast my cares on You, confident that You care for me [see 1 Peter 5:7].

DAY 7: *Reflections*

In the Chinese language, words are made up of a series of characters that combine to give the intended meaning. We often find ancient wisdom in the way Chinese characters are placed together. For example, the word "busy" comprises two characters: "heart" and "killing." This wisdom has been forgotten in our fast-paced society.

Not only have our physical hearts suffered from the ill effects of business, such as stress, poor diet and lack of exercise, but our spiritual hearts have also suffered. When we allow ourselves to constantly rush around trying to get this or that done, we kill something vital in ourselves; we smother the quiet wisdom of our heart. Succumbing to our society's "more is better" motto causes us to become impatient with ourselves—and with others. We miss the presence of God that surrounds us and brings us joy and peace. Unpracticed in the art of quiet, we hope to find our safety, our belonging and our healing by increasing our levels of accomplishment. But if inner peace were achieved through accomplishment, we would not still be striving. Peace would have been ours years ago. Rather, we must learn to appreciate the millions of quiet moments that nourish and refresh our soul.

First Place helps us learn to quit killing our hearts! Instead of filling our lives with busyness that does not leave time for personal care, we eat a balanced diet that is low in fat, cholesterol and salt by following the Live-It plan. We exercise three to five times a week to keep our heart fit, and we spend quiet time each day so that our priorities are in line with God's will. By memorizing Scripture, we hide God's Word in our hearts so that we have a shield of protective joy and peace to guard our hearts and minds. Our daily Bible study and Scripture reading reinforce our commitment to care for our hearts by affirming our importance to God and His unconditional love, neither of which depend on our accomplishments.

God invites us to quit killing our hearts and to find our peace, safety, belonging and healing in Him. Through diligent application of the Nine Commitments of First Place, we will have healthy hearts that please God.

Thank You, Lord, for being my peace. I know that a peaceful heart gives life to my body [see Proverbs 14:30].

Gracious God, forgive me for the times I harm my body because I refuse to find my rest in You.

Sovereign Lord, through the power of Your Holy Spirit, give me the grace to serve You with zeal and spiritual fervor so that I will not give in to fatigue and frustration as I endeavor to do the work You have set before me.

GROUP PRAYER REQUESTS   TODAY'S DATE:_____

NAME	REQUEST	RESULTS

SECURE THE HEARTLAND

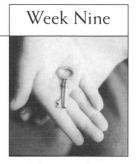

MEMORY VERSE
Above all else, guard your heart,
for it is the wellspring of life.
Proverbs 4:23

The initial rebuilding phase is not the end of our restoration work. We will spend our whole lives maintaining the healthy bodies and intact boundaries for which we have labored. We must also post a continual guard to protect our work, because we live in a sinful world and are always vulnerable to the enemy's attacks. Like a watchman on the city wall, we must continually survey the horizon for signs of impending invasion. Sometimes our own foolish choices allow the enemy to worm his way back into our personal space.

Look at any map of the Jerusalem wall and you will see that the Temple sits in the most guarded and reinforced part of the city wall. As we have already learned, the Holy Spirit has taken up residence inside all who believe in Jesus as Savior and Lord. For this reason, guarding our hearts must be our first priority, for our heart is the temple of the Holy Spirit, the wellspring of our life (see Proverbs 4:23).

DAY 1: *Family Ties*

After 52 days of hard labor and perseverance in the face of great danger, the Israelites finished restoring the Jerusalem wall. God had indeed fought with and for the Jews as they laid brick upon brick in the midst of hostile threats. God's gracious hand was upon His people as they endeavored to do His will. Pause for a moment and picture their joy and renewed confidence in God's faithfulness and love, and their relief at having completed such a daunting task.

Another group of people, however, was not feeling victorious. Turn in your Bible to Nehemiah 6:15-16 and read about what happened to those who opposed the rebuilding effort.

≫ What had Nehemiah's enemies lost? Why?

What happened to the threats they had used in an attempt to intimidate the workers?

Yet even though God had shown Himself to be the mighty defender of His chosen people, there were many in Judah who continued to communicate with the enemy! The walls had been rebuilt and the gates were in place, yet the enemy still had an open channel into the city.

≫ Read Nehemiah 6:17-19 and summarize in your own words what was happening.

Unfortunately, this was not an isolated incident. Tobiah was given entrance into Jerusalem another time because of family ties.

≫ Turn to Nehemiah 13:4-9. Summarize how Eliashib the priest disobeyed God and helped Tobiah because they were related.

Guarding our hearts is very important. This is a difficult concept for many of us to grasp fully, but we need to seriously evaluate whom we interact with on a daily basis.

⋙ Reflect on those you continue to associate with even though they might undermine God's good work in your life. Make a list of people (and things) you continue to invite into your life even though they might put you at risk.

⋙ According to Proverbs 25:26, what will happen to the wellspring of your life if you do not carefully guard this precious treasure from the people you listed?

On Day 5 of week five we looked at the cost of commitment. Recall Jesus' words in Luke 14:26. We must remain vigilant and make sure others do not pollute our personal space or divert us from our primary purpose: wholeheartedly serving God. We belong to the family of God; those who do God's will are our relatives (see Mark 3:35). We are called to pray for those outside the family of faith, but we cannot allow them to undermine our devotion to our Lord and Savior.

⋙ What do you need to do today to protect yourself from the people or things that Satan might use to pollute your personal space?

As you evaluate the people with whom you interact every day, listen closely for God's voice on the matter and trust that He will give you the strength you need to follow through.

 Lord God, Your gracious hand has been upon me and You have given me success. Help me not to pollute what You have called holy by allowing unhealthy people into my personal space.

Sovereign Lord, help me guard my heart, for it is the wellspring of life and the temple of Your Holy Spirit [see Proverbs 4:23].

DAY 2: *Gatekeepers*

After the walls had been rebuilt and the door set in place, Nehemiah took measures to ensure the future safety of the residents of Jerusalem.

➤ According to Nehemiah 7:1-3, what individuals and groups of people did Nehemiah appoint to protect Jerusalem's integrity?

Recall from week three that the gates were there to allow friendly people and needed supplies into the city and to keep hostile forces out. Gates also allowed the people to share the good things inside the city with others and to dispose of refuse and other things that might contaminate the city. The gatekeepers whom Nehemiah appointed had the important job of monitoring who and what passed in and out of the city walls.

As you learned in Wellness Worksheet One, we have both internal and external boundaries. The external boundaries are visible barriers, much like the city gates, that protect our private space. Internal boundaries are invisible walls that control what comes in and goes out. Another phrase for internal boundaries is self-control.

➤ Why are both external and internal boundaries necessary for the protection of your inner space?

➤ Reread Nehemiah 7:2. What are we told about Hananiah, the man Nehemiah put in charge of Jerusalem?

A practical definition of the word "integrity" is doing the right thing even though no one is looking.

≫ Turn in your Bible to Psalm 139:1-12 and prayerfully read David's words. Is there ever a time when God is not looking?

For those who believe in the sovereignty of God, integrity might be better described as doing the right thing because God is always looking!

≫ How is personal integrity part of your internal boundary system? Do you make healthy choices because you know God is always looking and sees even those things you do in secret? Explain your answer.

 All-seeing God, You are familiar with everything I do and say [see Psalm 139:3]. Help me do what is pleasing in Your sight. Sovereign Lord, I praise You because I am wonderfully made. I will protect and care for my body because Your works are wonderful [see Psalm 139:14].

DAY 3: *Sentries and Singers*

Refer to the list you made yesterday of the groups and individuals Nehemiah appointed to protect Jerusalem and govern the people. In addition to gate-keepers and overseers, Nehemiah appointed Levites to regulate Temple worship.

≫ According to verse 1, what other type of people did Nehemiah appoint?

At first glance, they may seem out of place in this list of guards and governors. But think back to another time when we saw singers appointed as part of Israel's defense.

≫ What was the occasion? (If necessary, turn back to Day 3 of week five to help you answer this question.)

≫ What happened as a result of the songs of praise that preceded the Israelite army?

Just as praise and victory are connected, singing praises to God is also linked with our protection! To better understand this connection, turn to 2 Chronicles 5:11-14.

≫ What happened in the Temple while the singers and musicians were praising God?

≫ Combine that illustration with Paul's words in Philippians 4:4-5. What happens when we rejoice?

Do you remember the words of Psalm 8:2 from our earlier studies? Praise silences the foe and the avenger. When God is in our midst, we shall not fall (see Psalm 46:5).

≫ Since learning about the powerful effects of singing God's praises in week five, have you incorporated more praise into your life? What new blessings have you discovered as a result of your songs of praise?

When we praise God, He fills the temples of our hearts and guards us with His presence.

 Integrity and uprightness will protect me because my hope is in You, O Lord, God of hosts [see Psalm 25:21].

Almighty God, You will rescue me because I love You. You will protect me because I acknowledge Your name [see Psalm 91:14].

DAY 4: God's Limits

Often we think of limits negatively, but in God's kingdom, limits protect us and define us as His people. Having appointed gatekeepers, singers, Levites and governors, Nehemiah gave the people some limitations.

≫ Summarize the limitations Nehemiah gave the people, as recorded in Nehemiah 7:3.

Since the beginning of creation, men and women have resisted God's limitations and seen the commandments that God gave them for their protection as something to rebel against. God defines limitations differently.

≫ Read Deuteronomy 4:5-8. What did God tell His people about His commandments through His servant Moses?

≫ What did God's righteous decrees prove to the other nations?

What was the source of Israel's greatness?

As much as we resist God's commandments and righteous decrees (i.e., limitations), God tells us they define us as His people. He is near us when we pray to Him because we are a people defined by His commandments.

≫ For review, what did you learn yesterday about God's being near?

Explain why accepting God's limitations—obeying His commands and decrees—is part of praising God.

≫ How do the limitations of the First Place program contribute to your protection system?

If God gives us limitations as a sign of His love and protection, why do you continue to resist them?

Most of us resist God's limitations because the negative voices in our head tell us God is cruel and punitive. We see Him as a parent who enforces needless restrictions. Ironically, we resist God's protection and yet embrace the harmful things of the world.

⤜ What thoughts do you need to bring captive to the Word of God so that you can change your attitude about staying within God's limitations?

 O Lord, I will walk about in freedom, for I have chosen to stay within the limitations You have given me for my protection [see Psalm 119:45].

Gracious God, teach me to obey Your commands, for there I find delight [see Psalm 119:35].

DAY 5: Healthy Outlets

Much of our study on boundaries has focused on keeping out the bad, however, healthy boundaries not only keep out harmful elements, but they also allow us to dispose of internal toxins in a healthy way, thus keeping them from polluting our personal space.

There was no plumbing in ancient cities. Refuse and trash had to be removed from the city. Burial grounds were also outside the city walls, as were quarantine spaces for people with infectious diseases.

⤜ Read Matthew 12:33-37 and Matthew 15:16-20. What valuable lessons did Jesus teach in these passages?

⤜ What do these lessons teach?

Just as we must find healthy ways to deal with physical refuse and trash that threaten to pollute our environment, so we must also find healthy ways to dispose of the negative thoughts and emotions that reside within us and threaten our internal security. We would never think of dumping our trash in our neighbor's living room. Instead of carelessly littering, we dispose of trash properly. Likewise, we should never spew our vile emotions onto others, or let them throw their emotional garbage into our space. We must all dispose of our inevitable pent-up emotions in appropriate ways. Writing in your journal is an excellent way to diffuse negative emotions, so is vigorous physical exercise.

➤ List several other healthy, God-honoring ways you can deal with hostile thoughts and feelings.

Did you list crying out to God in your anger and pain and asking Him to fill you with His love and peace? How about asking for forgiveness and allowing God to wash away your sins?

If we are willing to let Him, Jesus can transform our inner bitterness by the indwelling presence of His Holy Spirit. Exodus 15:22-25 recounts a time when the Israelites came to water that was too bitter to drink.

➤ What did Moses do to make the water sweet?

That piece of wood reminds us of the wooden cross on Calvary, where Jesus died so that your life can be transformed from bitter to sweet. Write a prayer thanking God for sending Jesus to die so that your life can be transformed into the temple of His Holy Spirit.

If you find yourself unable to control your negative thoughts and toxic emotions, you may need to talk to your pastor or a professional Christian counselor. He or she can help you find healthy ways to deal with the poison inside that threatens your safety and security. Remember, you may not be responsible for the things that caused the bitterness and pain, but you are responsible for dealing with the problem in a mature,

Christian way that brings honor and glory to God. Ignoring or denying the pain only compounds the problem. You will need to be strong and courageous as you face the root cause of the distress, but God is with you and will help you if you are willing to cry out to Him for help.

I will sing to the Lord a new song and praise His name, for He has done marvelous things in my life [see Psalm 98:1].

O Lord my God, you have turned my wailing into dancing and clothed me with joy [see Psalm 30:11].

DAY 6: *Reflections*

When most of us contemplate evil, we conjure up visions of fierce predators that pose imminent danger to our safety and security. However, we must never discount the wiles of the evil one. He is cunning and crafty. He will not send a roaring lion when a cute little fox will serve his purpose. That is why Solomon admonishes us to catch the little foxes that nibble away at the tender vines, destroying the crop before it can develop (see Song of Songs 2:15). The little foxes in our lives are usually the petty annoyances that keep us from focusing on the one important thing—our relationship with God. Little foxes erode our peace and serenity and keep us distracted and frustrated. Often, the seemingly innocent little animals are the daily irritations and anxieties we tolerate instead of taking definite action to ban them from our spiritual garden.

Catching the little foxes is an important concept for First Place participants. Satan easily persuades us that the little things we do that keep us from following the Nine Commitments of First Place aren't a big deal, but they end up gobbling up our time and leave us feeling frustrated and ineffective. When the foxes run unchecked, they prevent us from keeping the Nine Commitments. At the end of the day, we stare at a Commitment Record with unchecked boxes and wonder where the time went. Perhaps we are even reluctant to attend our weekly First Place meeting because we have nothing to share with the group. We feel like a failure for having not kept the Nine Commitments that week, when our real failure was not realizing what great damage those pesky little foxes can do!

We must capture those little pests that have nibbled away at our commitments and kept them from being fruitful. Take time today to consider what little foxes you are allowing to nibble away at your time. Remember, all change begins with awareness.

 Lord, help me to catch the little foxes that nibble away at the vines and strip me of my joy and peace [see Song of Songs 2:15].
    Faithful Father, teach me knowledge and good judgment because I trust in your commands [see Psalm 119:66].
    Gracious God, thank You for Your Word and Your truth.

DAY 7: *Reflections*

Many of us grew up believing that anger is a sin, yet nothing could be further from the truth. Anger is a natural human emotion, and to get angry is not a sin. Anger is a valuable emotion that can tell us when our boundaries have been violated and we are in danger. God has given us this emotion as part of our protection system; a signal to alert us when our safety and well-being are threatened. That said, we must learn to deal with our anger in appropriate ways. We need to find safe outlets for our anger and frustration.

This volatile emotion can be frightening to those of us who were taught that expressing anger is wrong. As a result, we let it build up way beyond healthy limits and then are shocked when it comes out in inappropriate ways. When we deny our anger we ignore an emotional boundary God has given us for our protection. Hiding our anger is not an acceptable solution either. We are to handle this God-given emotion in God's way. How? God says, "In your anger do not sin; when you are on your beds, search your hearts and be silent" (Psalm 4:4). First Place gives us the tools we need to deal with repressed anger so that it no longer damages ourselves, others or our relationships with God.

Many of us learned as children to deal with anger by stuffing it down with excess food. As we begin practicing the Live-It plan and stop suppressing our anger with food, we discover a smoldering inferno inside us—a literal fire in the belly. What we identified before as heartburn from overeating, we now recognize as repressed anger eating away at our insides. The exercise commitment of First Place provides us with a safe outlet for our anger. When we feel tension building up, we can take a break and go for a walk. Perhaps we need to aggressively work out our anger through kickboxing or some other vigorous aerobic activity, done in a controlled environment that does not produce injury to self or others. At other times we may need to go to a deserted place and cry out to the Lord in prayer. Whatever the outlet, we can learn to recognize anger as a God-given emotion and learn healthy ways to release it within the boundaries of the First Place program. We can be on fire for the Lord, but we don't need to suffer from fire in the belly now that we are practicing the Nine Commitments of First Place.

Father, anger can be a frightening emotion. Help me find healthy ways to relieve the tension in my life so that I will not use my anger as an excuse to sin.

Listen to my prayer, O God, hear me and answer me [see Psalm 55:1].

Lord, You call me to guard my heart because it is the temple where Your Holy Spirit resides. Help me to be obedient to Your command and diligently guard myself against those who threaten to pollute what You have made clean.

GROUP PRAYER REQUESTS   TODAY'S DATE:_____

NAME	REQUEST	RESULTS

RECLAIM GOD'S PROMISES

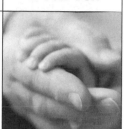

MEMORY VERSE

Then a cloud appeared and enveloped them,
and a voice came from the cloud:
"This is my Son, whom I love. Listen to him!"

Mark 9:7

In week one, we learned that Jesus is the truth who came to set us free.
We looked to the truth of God's Word as we began to build healthy
boundaries that allow us to live lives wholeheartedly devoted to God. We
struggled along with Nehemiah and his band of workers as they restored
the walls and gates of Jerusalem so that the Israelites could live in safety
and peace. In reading their story, we found courage to restore the inner
boundaries in our own lives that have been crumbled and charred by hostile forces. We have done the work—now it is time to reap the benefits of
our labors! This week we will focus on our responsibilities as those who
have been set free: to worship God and to be ambassadors of reconciliation as He works to redeem a lost and fallen world.

DAY 1: *Free to Worship God*

Nehemiah 7 ends with a statement of victory: "The priests, the Levites,
the gatekeepers, the singers and the temple servants, along with certain
of the people and the rest of the Israelites, settled in their own towns"
(Nehemiah 7:73). The walls and gates had been restored, and the Temple
and town had been put in order. The Israelites were free from the threat
of invasion and could live in safety and security. However, they lacked
one thing in response: a time of worship and celebration.

How easily Satan dupes us into believing we have been set free so
that we can live lives of ease and comfort. Self-serving freedom is just another of Satan's subtle lies. When the Israelites were in cruel bondage to

the Egyptians, God sent Moses to deliver them from the hand of oppression, but God never intended to set them free to do their own thing!

➣ According to Exodus 3:18 and Exodus 8:1, for what purpose did Moses ask Pharaoh to set the people free?

Exodus 6:2-8 contains God's words to Moses prior to the deliverance. Read that passage prayerfully, and then answer the following questions:

➣ God made a covenant promise to Abraham, Isaac and Jacob. What did God promise to give them (v. 4)?

➣ What had gotten God's attention? What did God remember as a result (v. 5)?

➣ Summarize the words God gave Moses to say to the Israelites.

What an amazing promise! God would free the Israelites and redeem them from bondage. He would take them as His own people and He would be their God! Verse 8 ends with the assurance, "I am the Lord."

➣ Now read Exodus 6:9. What happened when Moses related God's promise of deliverance to the people?

What kept them from hearing God's words?

As long as we are enslaved and in bondage we are not free to listen to God and worship Him with wholehearted devotion. End today's lesson with a reflective time as you ask yourself this possibly piercing question: What keeps me discouraged and in cruel bondage so that I cannot listen to God and worship Him? Be sure to include the things that keep you from fully committing to the First Place program, for the program is part of God's will for your life. Record in the space provided or in your journal the hindrances that come to mind.

Lord God Almighty, when the Son sets me free I will be free indeed [see John 8:36]. Lord, I want to use my freedom to worship and listen to You.

God, I know that Your Word is truth. Help me listen to every word You speak as You sanctify me by Your truth [see John 17:17].

DAY 2: *Free to Listen to His Voice*

Two men were walking along a crowded city sidewalk. Suddenly one of them remarked, "Listen to the sound of the cricket!" But his friend, who had not trained himself to listen to the sounds of nature, could not hear the cricket above the roar of the traffic and the sounds of the people scurrying around.

So it is with hearing God speak. We must learn to listen, training ourselves to hear His voice above the noise and confusion of the world. We must learn to tune out the cacophony of voices that vie for our attention and pay close attention to God's words.

As the Israelites prepared to enter the Promised Land, Moses laid down some final instructions. Moses would not be making the final leg of the journey with them, and he issued them a stern warning. Read his words in Deuteronomy 30:19-20 out loud so that you can hear your own voice reciting these important truths.

≫ What were the Israelites to do? Why?

≫ Verse 20 tells us that the Lord is our_____. What do you choose when you refuse to listen to God's voice?

Listening to God's voice is not an Old Testament concept that does not apply to New Testament Christians. Jesus told His followers there was a group of people who would listen to His voice.

≫ Turn to John 10:1-18. In your own words, explain who recognizes Jesus' voice and listens to Him.

In Revelation 2—3, God gave a message to seven churches. Although these seven churches were literal churches, most Bible scholars agree that they symbolically represent the Church and believers in the current age.

≫ What words do Revelation 2:7,11,17,29 and 3:6,13,22 have in common?

He who has an_____, let him_____what the_____

says to the_____.

➢ From our studies in week one, Day 1, what is one of the many things the Spirit does in the lives of believers?

➢ Summarize what you have learned today about the importance of listening to God's voice.

How does this week's memory verse confirm your findings?

 Loving Father, thank You for sending the Holy Spirit to guide me into all truth [see John 16:13]. Give me ears to hear what He is saying to me through my daily Bible study and prayer.
   Lord, Your words are truth and life. Help me to listen to Your voice and hold fast to Your commands [see Deuteronomy 30:20].

DAY 3: *Free to Worship*

As you begin today's lesson, take time to read Nehemiah 8. After the walls had been rebuilt and the people had settled in their towns, they all assembled for a specific purpose.

➢ For what purpose did the people assemble (vv. 1-2)?

➤ Reread verse 3 and then fill in the blanks.

And_____the people_____attentively to the_____.

➤ What did the people do as a result (v. 6)?

As a result of listening to the Word of God and praising Him in worship, something else happened to the people.

➤ According to verse 9, what else were the people doing? Why do you think they did this?

When we hear God's Word with understanding and worship Him with praise, we should always be convicted of our sinful condition. The people realized they had not been keeping God's law or giving Him the praise He deserved.

➤ According to Proverbs 1:7, what is the beginning of knowledge?

To fear God does not mean to be afraid of Him, it means to revere and respect Him because of who He is and what He has done for His people.

➤ How is listening to God's voice an important part of fearing Him?

➢ Nehemiah told the people not to grieve and weep; they were to celebrate. Carefully read Nehemiah 8:9-12 and explain the reason for their celebration.

Hearing God's Word with new ears and understanding what has been revealed to us is always a reason for great joy!

➢ What new things has God revealed to You through His Word in this Bible study?

We have learned in previous lessons that singing God's praises is essential to victory and protection.

➢ Reread Nehemiah 8:10. Combining Nehemiah's words with the principles you have learned about praise, what conclusion can you draw about the joy of the Lord?

Spend time praising God for giving you ears to hear and a willingness to listen to His voice. Write a brief psalm of praise in the space below.

Almighty God, I will rejoice because You are my strength and my song.

Gracious Father, Your statutes are my delight and my counselors [see Psalm 119:24]. Thank You for Your Word and for giving me new understanding of what it means to praise Your holy name in worship.

DAY 4: *Free to Hear the Cries of the Poor*

Throughout salvation history, God has presented Himself as the defender of widows, orphans, aliens and the poor. Many of God's commands deal with the fair treatment of these people, and He gave the Israelites special laws to protect the poorest of the poor from financial oppression and tyranny.

Our praises can never please God while we ignore the cries of the poor and the oppressed. Turn to Isaiah 58 to read about worship that pleases God.

➤ What do we have to do in order to be called a "Repairer of Broken Walls" and "Restorer of Streets with Dwellings" (vv. 9-12)? Summarize God's message contained in these verses.

➤ According to verses 6 through 9, what kind of worship pleases God? Listen to God's voice while summarizing these verses in your own words.

➤ What will happen if we listen to God's Word and consider the needs of the poor and oppressed? Write verse 14 below, exactly as it appears in your Bible.

Yesterday we saw another verse with the words "the joy of the Lord." Reread Nehemiah 8:10.

➤ What conclusion do you draw by comparing Isaiah 58 with Nehemiah 8:10?

With which specific group of people were the worshipers to share their celebration and feasting?

We cannot expect to find joy in the Lord, or to claim Him as our source of strength, if we are mistreating others and not responsive to the cries of the poor. Before we engage in worship and praise, we must be sure we are treating others with the same mercy and compassion God has shown us.

Who are the spiritually poor and oppressed with whom you need to share the blessings of First Place? Make a list and take time to share your joy in the Lord with at least one of these people today

 Lord, You care about the needs of Your people. Allow me to be a channel of blessing to hurting individuals.
Gracious God, when I listen to Your voice, You make my joy complete [see Deuteronomy 16:15].

DAY 5: *Free to Hear and Do*

No matter how carefully we listen to God's voice, unless we put His words into practice, we can never fully experience God's will for our lives. God's Word only has life-changing power when we actually practice it.

Jesus told a parable about two builders: one wise and one foolish. Read this familiar story found in Matthew 7:24-27.

What distinguished the wise builder from the foolish builder?

✳ Complete the following sentence:

Everyone who hears these words of mine and_____them into

_____is like a wise man who built his house on the

rock (v. 24).

✳ Referring to our studies in week four, who is our rock?

✳ How is listening to Jesus' words and putting them into practice like building on a solid foundation?

✳ Now turn to Ephesians 2:20. What is the foundation we are to build on, and who is the chief cornerstone?

✳ Explain the analogy James uses in James 1:22-25 to describe those who hear God's Word but don't put it into practice.

What does James say we do when we merely listen to the word (v. 22)?

Jesus Christ is the way, the truth and the life. But in order to benefit from this indescribable gift, we must listen to what He says and put His words into practice.

➤ What words of Jesus are you refusing to listen to? Or having heard and understood, how are you deceiving yourself by not putting them into practice?

No matter how carefully we have rebuilt our inner boundaries, unless they are built on the rock, the Word of God made flesh, we have been foolish builders whose work will not survive the storms of life.

➤ From memory, write Mark 9:7 below.

Now commit yourself to obey the voice from the cloud that said, "This is my Son, whom I love. Listen to him!" Be sure to commit to all Nine Commitments of First Place as part of your commitment and your obedience to God. Write your commitment in the space provided.

 Sovereign Lord, all too often I hear Your voice and then go about my busy days unaffected by the words that have the power to transform my life. Help me to be a hearer and doer of Your Word of truth.

God of heaven and Earth, Your Word is my rock, my sure foundation, the source of my joy and my strength.

DAY 6: *Reflections*

Often we get so caught up in the spectacular miracles Jesus performed while here on Earth that we fail to see their significance in our everyday, not-so-spectacular lives. Think back to Jesus' first miracle, the miracle in which He turned ordinary water into sparkling wine at a wedding feast in Cana. What significance could that miracle possibly have in our lives today? The key is found in the simple words of Jesus' mother: "Do whatever he tells you" (John 2:5). Jesus used the willing obedience of the servants to transform the ordinary into the superb. God provided the divine, transforming power; the servants did the human footwork. Had they refused to fill the jars with water, there would have been no spectacular wine.

Like the servants at the wedding feast, we too need to be told, "Do whatever [Christ] tells you." If we are willing to cooperate with the process, Jesus can take our plain, ordinary, empty lives and transform them into something beautiful. Participation in First Place is about doing the footwork. As we fill the jars, we trust Jesus to perform the miracles. We do everything He tells us in faith, trusting He will display His divine, transforming power in and through us.

Are you willing to do everything He tells you? Are you ready to start today? He can transform your life and rebuild your shattered inner walls if you are willing to put brick upon brick and be part of the process.

 Lord Jesus, I am confident You can turn my ordinary life into a spectacular miracle if I am willing to hear Your words and do everything You tell me to do.

Gracious God, Your Word lights my path so that my feet won't stumble [see Psalm 119:105]. Give me the strength to follow You and be obedient to Your commands.

Precious Lord, I will show my love for You by sitting at Your feet and listening to Your words.

DAY 7: *Reflections*

Today marks the last lesson of this Bible study. We have read God's Word and been given new eyes and a fresh understanding of His truth. Many of the lessons have been difficult to hear, and even more difficult to put into practice. Yet unless we read, hear and take His words to heart, we cannot live lives that please God—lives marked by joy, peace and security.

Take a few moments to mentally review the things you have learned during our 10-week study. Make a list below of the most important and memorable principles you have learned.

Now ask yourself how you can continue to put these lessons into practice to maintain the boundary walls you have worked so hard to build. (Quiet time with God—daily time spent listening for your master's voice— will be vital as you go from here. The voice from the cloud didn't say, "This is my Son, do something productive for Him." God said, "This is my Son . . . Listen to him." What is He saying to you today?

 Today I have heard Your voice and I will not harden my heart. I will bow down in worship because You are the Lord, my maker [see Psalm 95:6-8].

Great God and King, You are above all gods. I will sing for joy to You, O Lord, for You are my rock and my salvation [see Psalm 95:1-3].

Almighty God, You have shown me such grace because I have listened to Your words and put them into practice. Thank You for including me in Your family and for giving me the Holy Spirit to help me accomplish Your work here on Earth.

GROUP PRAYER REQUESTS   TODAY'S DATE:_____

NAME	REQUEST	RESULTS

Do not move an ancient boundary stone.
Proverbs 23:10

When most of us hear the term "boundaries," we immediately think of a fence or wall, set up to define property lines and keep out unwanted intruders. Certainly physical boundaries are the easiest to see and define. No matter the form, all physical boundaries convey the same message: This is where my property begins—respect that.

The concept of boundaries comes from the very nature of God. In His Word, God defines Himself, takes responsibility for His actions and communicates with us about His plans, His feelings and His desires for His people. God is separate and holy, and He calls us to set ourselves apart as holy unto Him.

There are many types of physical boundaries. For example, skin defines who we are and where others stop and we begin. Another physical boundary we often overlook is money. We keep our funds in separate accounts so that they don't commingle with those of other bank patrons, and wallets and safes protect our financial reserves.

➤ Take a few moments to write down a few other physical boundaries that define property lines and give ownership and responsibility.

In the mental, emotional and spiritual realms, boundaries are every bit as important as physical boundaries, but much more difficult to see and define. By recognizing and defining our invisible boundaries, we can take ownership for what goes on inside our own skin. Internal boundaries allow us to take ownership and give us the freedom to live without the threat of harmful forces that threaten our safety and security. Internal boundaries allow us to take responsibility for our own actions. They also allow us to be responsible to God for the way we manage our life in relation to His God-given limitations and boundaries. Another word for internal boundaries is "self-control."

God's Word clearly defines our boundaries and gives us limitations for our protection. When we don't understand what these internal boundaries are, or how to defend them, we allow others to intrude into our space and keep us from living lives holy and set apart for God.

Let's take some time to talk more in-depth about each of these three internal boundary categories, beginning with mental boundaries.

MENTAL BOUNDARIES

Mental boundaries allow us to think our own thoughts and form our own opinions while being able to reject the thoughts and opinions of others that run contrary to our belief system. Mental boundaries give us the freedom to think for ourselves and then to express those thoughts in appropriate ways. Have you ever started talking and then had someone else finish your sentence for you? That was an invasion of your mental boundaries. Only God can know your inner thoughts. Have you ever been told, "I know what you are thinking," or said that to someone else? That too violates mental boundaries. Someone without healthy emotional boundaries could be described as a chameleon—the person takes on the thoughts and opinions of whomever he or she is with at the moment. Forcing our opinions on another is also a violation of his or her mental boundaries; we can share our opinions, but we should never force others to accept them.

≫ List several unseen mental boundaries that God has established for your protection.

EMOTIONAL BOUNDARIES

Emotional boundaries allow us to have our own feelings and express them in appropriate ways. Healthy emotional boundaries keep us from taking on the emotions of others and from imposing our emotions on them. People with damaged emotional boundaries spew their emotional garbage all over anyone who will listen, and try to manipulate others through guilt, shame and fear.

➣ Make a list of several emotional boundaries that you need to protect as diligently as you protect the physical boundaries that define your physical property lines.

SPIRITUAL BOUNDARIES

Spiritual boundaries define our concept of God and keep us separate from God, who calls us to relationship, not oneness, with Him. When our spiritual boundaries are damaged, we continually vie with God for power and try to play God in the lives of others.

Healthy spiritual boundaries allow us to hear God's voice and respond without interference from others who take their direction from another master. They also allow us to cling to our personal relationship with God, even when others try to impose their false beliefs on us.

➣ Make a list of spiritual boundaries that define who you are in relation to God, remembering that God calls His people to be holy and separate.

IDENTIFYING UNHEALTHY BOUNDARIES

If we had healthy, intact boundaries we would not be doing this Bible study or participating in First Place! The very fact that we cannot control what we eat indicates that our boundaries are damaged and in need of rebuilding. We put food into our mouths (which are part of our physical boundary systems), even though it can damage our bodies. We pollute our own space!

Described below are three degrees of damaged boundaries, followed by a description of healthy boundaries. No matter how damaged your boundaries are now, God calls you to rebuild them so that you can be holy and set apart for Him. What He asks you to do, He also equips you to do. Courageously look at the types of boundaries so that you can accurately assess your situation.

DAMAGED BOUNDARIES

Having damaged boundaries is like living in a room with intact walls and a solid door—but the doorknob is on the outside. Other people have permission to control what comes in and what goes out of our personal space.

Those of us with damaged boundaries take on responsibilities, thoughts and feelings that are not ours. We are not sure where we stop and others begin. The number of people who have access to our personal space depends on the degree of damage; but no matter how severe, our damaged boundaries keep us from controlling what goes on inside our own skin. Outside forces have the ability to enter in unhindered and throw us off course.

COLLAPSED BOUNDARIES

Having collapsed boundaries is like living without any protection.

This is the most severe type of boundary damage. Our walls are crumbled, and there are no doors. Hostile raiding parties come and go at will. No matter how good our intentions, outside forces keep us from living a life of direction and purpose.

Collapsed boundaries are marked by excess—too much goes out and too much comes in. Not only are we not in control, but also we can't even define what we are supposed to control. We have no property lines or boundaries to keep out unwanted forces.

Binge eating, physical abuse (giving or receiving), compulsive spending and sexual promiscuity are all indicators of collapsed boundaries.

WALLED BOUNDARIES

Nothing comes in and nothing goes out of walled boundaries. We live in a room that has thick walls with no doors or windows.

Walled boundaries result in loneliness, isolation, stagnation and emotional starvation. Often we erect this type of boundary as a result of fear, doubt and suspicion based on past scarring and fear of future negative interaction with others. We become emotionally unavailable and turn to food and other substances for comfort because they do not pose a threat to our security. Walled boundaries often manifest themselves as a wall of body fat that insulates the frightened child inside and gives us a false sense of security.

HEALTHY BOUNDARIES

Having healthy boundaries is like living in a room with intact walls and a solid door that has a doorknob only on the inside.

Healthy boundaries allow us to determine what comes in and what goes out of our lives. We are open and receptive to others, but we can selectively reject those things that threaten our internal security. For those of us who are serious about our relationship with God, healthy boundaries help us keep out people, thoughts, emotions and beliefs that interfere with our commitment to God. Healthy boundaries allow us to set goals and keep out the things that divert us from achieving results.

ASSESSING YOUR BOUNDARIES

Now it is time to apply what we have learned. Please be honest as you do this assessment. We cannot begin to repair something until we acknowledge it is broken. You may have stronger boundaries in some areas than in others, but unless all your boundary categories are healthy, you need to go through the rebuilding process.

➣ Based on the four boundary categories we just discussed, which term best illustrates the condition of your personal boundaries?

☐ Collapsed   ☐ Healthy

☐ Damaged   ☐ Walled

PHYSICAL BOUNDARIES

Place a Y for "yes" or an N for "no" next to each of the following statements.

Are you in control of what comes in and out of your physical space?

_____

Can you let in the good and let out both the bad and the good with prudent discretion?_____

Do you allow others to impose themselves on you physically?_____

Are you a good steward of your money and control what goes out and comes into your financial house?_____

Are you able to control your physical desires for intimacy, keeping yourself sexually pure?_____

➤ Briefly describe any other physical boundary issues you feel are pertinent to evaluating your boundary health.

➤ On a scale of 1 to 10, rate the health of your physical boundaries.

1	2	3	4	5	6	7	8	9	10

Severe Damage   Optimal Boundary Health

MENTAL BOUNDARIES

Place a Y for "yes" or an N for "no" next to each of the following statements.

Do you feel you are entitled to your own thoughts and opinions?

_____

Can you express your thoughts and opinions openly, without fear of rejection?_____

Do you allow others to impose their thoughts and opinions on you?

_____

If you were to disagree with your spouse or a close friend on a political or social issue, could you agree to disagree and still be in relationship with that person? _____

Do you imagine you can tell what others are thinking, or that they know what you are thinking before you tell them? _____

➤ Briefly describe any other mental boundary issues you feel are pertinent to evaluating your boundary health.

➤ On a scale of 1 to 10, rate the health of your mental boundaries.

| 1 | 2 | 3 | 4 | 5 | 6 | 7 | 8 | 9 | 10 |

Severe Damage   Optimal Boundary Health

EMOTIONAL BOUNDARIES

Place a Y for "yes" or an N for "no" next to each of the following statements.

Do you take on the emotions of others or expect them to be responsible for your emotional stability?_____

Can you control your own emotions and express them appropriately? _____

Do you require others to control their emotions and express them appropriately?_____

Do you feel you are an emotional dumping ground where others are allowed to dispose of unhealthy emotions inappropriately? _____

Do you blame others for your moods or allow others to blame you for theirs?_____

Do you do things contrary to your belief system because you are afraid of hurting someone else's feelings?_____

Do you feel responsible for keeping others happy? _____

➤ Briefly describe any other emotional boundary issues you feel are pertinent to evaluating your boundary health.

➤ On a scale of 1 to 10, rate the health of your emotional boundaries.

| 1 | 2 | 3 | 4 | 5 | 6 | 7 | 8 | 9 | 10 |

Severe Damage   Optimal Boundary Health

SPIRITUAL BOUNDARIES

Place a Y for "yes" or an N for "no" next to each of the following statements.

Do you know where you stop and God begins? _____

Can you differentiate between God's responsibilities and yours?_____

Do you play God in others' lives by trying to save or rescue them instead of pointing them to the only One who can save?_____

Are you easily confused by false teachings or enticed by in vogue religious fads?_____

Are you firmly anchored in the Word of God?_____

Do you allow others—or negative voices in your own head—to tell you things about God that are contrary to His Word?_____

➤ Briefly describe any other spiritual boundary issues you feel are pertinent to evaluating your boundary health.

➤ On a scale of 1 to 10, rate the health of your spiritual boundaries.

| 1 | 2 | 3 | 4 | 5 | 6 | 7 | 8 | 9 | 10 |

Severe Damage   Optimal Boundary Health

Written Evaluation

Having completed your assessment, prepare a State of the Union report. Be sure to include your motivation for rebuilding. You will be sharing this report with your First Place group during week three.

Before sharing your report with your group, commit your findings to God and ask for His help. Listen for any special instruction He gives you during this quiet time. Your prayer journal is an excellent place to record that conversation.

End your assessment in prayer, asking for God's help and guidance as you begin the boundary-rebuilding project. Remember, there is no hurt He can't heal, no brokenness He can't repair. Let the healer of your soul hold you in His loving arms as you walk through this dark valley on your way to higher ground.

TIME ON YOUR SIDE

There is a time for everything, and a season for every activity under heaven.
Ecclesiastes 3:1

Time is also a God-given limitation, or boundary. No matter what we do, we cannot produce more than 24 hours in a day. We cannot beg, borrow or steal one second more, and unlike the popular "rollover minutes" offered in some wireless phone plans, we cannot save our unused minutes for future use.

Healthy time boundaries allow us to focus on the most important tasks of each moment, knowing there will be enough time to do everything God has called us to do. If we hear ourselves saying, "I just don't have enough time," we are likely taking on something God has not asked of us. God would have given us more than 24 hours each day if He felt we could not accomplish our God-given responsibilities within that time frame. Not having enough time is the result of taking on time commitments outside God's will for us.

Time is also a way of separating the past, present and future. Jesus told His disciples not to be concerned about tomorrow, for every day has enough trouble of its own (see Matthew 6:34). In First Place we keep a Commitment Record to keep track of our daily progress with the Nine Commitments. Food exchanges not used today cannot be saved for tomorrow. Exercise done yesterday isn't put in today's square. We don't do all our daily Bible studies in one setting; we do one study each day.

Take a few moments to reflect on how you can use time as a boundary. Maybe you need to set a time to get away and rest—a time away from activity so that you can hear God's voice in new and exciting ways. Maybe you need to take a "time out" from the forces that keep you off balance. Perhaps you need to limit the amount of time you expend on a given task or limit interaction with those who do not respect your time.

➤ List several ways you can incorporate time boundaries into your life.

Now look at your schedule and your calendar. This is a time to listen to Jesus and get your priorities straight.

➤ Do you consistently run short on time to accomplish all that you have heaped onto your plate?

If you answered yes to the previous question, perhaps you are devoting time to projects that will impress others but are not pleasing to God.

➤ Are you self-controlled with your time or do others dictate your priorities? Explain using specific examples.

➤ Go back to the house drawings in Wellness Worksheet One. Which drawing best describes the state of your time boundaries: damaged, collapsed, walled or healthy?

➤ Write a short report on the state of your time boundaries. Include several ways that you can begin rebuilding these boundaries today.

TEMPORARY
BOUNDARIES

You hem me in—behind and before.
Psalm 139:5

As you have learned from the previous Wellness Worksheets, we need
both external and internal boundaries. External boundaries are fixed lines
that keep us hemmed in, like a fenced yard that keeps a young child from
running into the street. Not all external boundaries are visible, but external boundaries are easy to define and defend. An external boundary might
be not frequenting a certain restaurant because when you go there you
always overeat.

External boundaries are best defined as self-control or integrity. Internal
boundaries allow us to do the right thing, even when no one else is looking. As a child grows and matures, he or she learns how to safely cross the
street, at which time the external fence boundary is no longer necessary.
After our internal boundary system has been rebuilt, we might be able to
go back to that favorite restaurant and stay within our Live-It plan.

External boundaries can act as "training boundaries," much like the
training wheels on a child's bicycle. Many times we need temporary external boundaries as restrictions that keep us in control until we have learned
to be self-controlled. During the early stages of recovery, these temporary
external boundaries keep us safe from forces that might overwhelm us. For
example, you may need to turn off the telephone during your quiet time
or limit the amount of time you spend with people who undermine your
goals. Another example would be cleaning out your cupboards to remove
any food outside the boundaries of your Live-It plan. Be creative in your
ideas.

➣ Make a list of at least 10 temporary external boundaries you will need
to establish while your internal boundary system is being repaired.

Now, using the triage concept (putting first things first), select one of those temporary external boundaries and put it in place today. No matter how great your list, your ideas will be for naught unless you establish these temporary boundaries and learn self-control.

FORGIVENESS AND RESTORATION

Forgive as the Lord forgave you.
Colossians 3:13

Above all else, guard your heart, for it is the wellspring of life.
Proverbs 4:23

As we discussed on Day 4 of week one, a paradox is a statement that appears to contradict itself but is really a truth applied to a deeper level of our being. Paradoxes may seem confusing when we try to interpret spiritual truth based on physical reality. This is certainly the case when we consider forgiveness and establishing healthy boundaries that keep us from being exposed to further harm. Scripture tells us to forgive those who have offended us (see Colossians 3:13) *and* to protect ourselves from future abuse (see Proverbs 4:23).

Those of us who have been the object of abuse are often hesitant to forgive our abusers because we fear forgiveness will open us up to future harm. But without appropriate boundaries, forgiving or not forgiving someone will not affect the outcome. Only proper boundaries can prevent continued abuse to ourselves or our loved ones, and forgiveness is a necessary step toward establishing healthy boundaries.

On Day 5 of week two (page 33) you made a list of those people whom you feel have injured you. Turn back to that list and write each name in the space below. To the right of each name write a short statement explaining how allowing that person back in your personal space might put you, or those entrusted to your care, in jeopardy.

Name	Risk of Future Harm

At this point you may be thinking, *I'm told to forgive these people, but they are a threat to my present security. Can that be what God wants for me?* The key to understanding this paradox is to understand the difference between forgiveness and restored relationships.

Forgiveness means giving up our right to get even and leaving vengeance to God (see Romans 12:19). Forgiveness is a unilateral decision. We choose to untie ourselves from past hurts rather than allow them to poison the present. Forgiveness is not dependent on the offender's response. As Christ's followers we forgive so that we can worship God unhindered by toxins that threaten to pollute what God has redeemed and called holy.

Restored relationships require both parties' involvement: One repents of the offense(s) committed and the other person forgives the offense(s). Take a moment to read Luke 3:8-14. Repentance is not about idle words. For restoration to take place, the offending party's repentance must manifest itself in changed behavior, and the fruit of repentance does not include continued abuse.

Damaged relationships can be restored in trust and safety when both parties accept mutual responsibility to each other and to the relationship. God calls us to forgive as He has forgiven us, but He also admonishes us to not open ourselves up to further abuse. Our Lord calls us to set limits to guard our physical, mental, emotional and spiritual property until the one who has violated our boundaries has repented and can be trusted again.

As Christians we need to associate with like-minded individuals who are willing to admit when they do something that has caused us harm. We're human too, and we also need to be aware and acknowledge when we hurt others. When we own up to our shortcomings, amend our behavior and strive to change, we learn through failure. We can forgive one another over and over again because both parties are committed to change and growth, and treat each other with dignity and respect. We can work through the problem together, restore the broken relationship and grow in the process.

➤ Write about a time when confession and repentance allowed you to safely forgive someone who had offended you.

How did you grow in your Christian walk as a result of that experience?

On the other hand, we need to avoid those people who deny that they have hurt us, who find various ways to justify their unacceptable behavior or who have no desire to treat us with love, respect and dignity now or in the future. A relationship with this type of person is destructive for all parties involved, and we must keep them at a safe distance. In extreme cases, we must avoid them altogether. Even though we have forgiven them from our hearts, we do not need to allow them back into our personal space.

Forgiveness gives us the freedom to set boundaries because it unhooks us from the hurtful person and allows us to act responsibly and wisely. Until we forgive, we are still tied in a destructive relationship with him or her. Unforgiveness destroys boundaries; forgiveness creates them. When we stop expecting to have a healthy relationship with an unhealthy person, we are free to establish relationships that nourish and support our

Christian maturity. This newfound freedom makes room for healthy relationships that contribute to our growth and healing and allow us to flourish.

Take time today to assess the quality of your relationships by mentally answering the following questions:

- Is there someone in your life with whom you continue to associate who repeatedly intrudes into your personal space and defiles what God has called you to keep holy and set apart for Him?

- Is there someone in your life who frequently shatters your plans and dreams?

- Is there someone in your life who sabotages your goals and tries to impose his or her thoughts and emotions on you?

- Is there someone in your life who promises to change but doesn't?

If so, you need to forgive that person, and then post a No Trespassing sign on the gate of your heart. Remember, God will not protect you if you do not take appropriate steps to protect yourself. We are not to put God to the test by allowing abusive people into our personal space.

➤ What action do you need to take today to forgive those who have hurt you *and* to take responsible action to protect your heart?

Write a prayer in your journal asking God to help you establish relationships founded on mutual respect and responsibility and to help you build healthy boundaries to protect you from those who continue to do you harm.

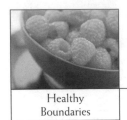

FIRST PLACE MENU PLANS

Each plan is based on approximately 1,400 calories.

Breakfast	0-1 meats, 1-2 breads, 1 fruit, 0-1 milk, 0-½ fat
Lunch	1-2 meats, 2 breads, 1 vegetable, 1 fruit, 1 fat
Dinner	2-3 meats, 2 breads, 2 vegetables, 1 fat
Snacks	1-2 breads, 1 fruit, 1 milk, ½ fat (or any remaining exchanges)
Daily Total	4-5 meats, 6-7 breads, 3-4 vegetables, 3-4 fruits, 2-3 milks, 3-4 fats

Note: You may always choose the high range for vegetables and fruits, but limit high range to only one category in meats, breads, milks or fats.

For more calories, add the following to the 1,400-calorie plan:

1,600 calories	2 breads, 1 fat
1,800 calories	2 meats, 3 breads, 1 vegetable, 1 fat
2,000 calories	2 meats, 4 breads, 1 vegetable, 3 fats
2,200 calories	2 meats, 5 breads, 1 vegetable, 1 fruit, 5 fats
2,400 calories	2 meats, 6 breads, 2 vegetables, 1 fruit, 6 fats

The exchanges for these meals were calculated using the MasterCook software. It uses a database of over 6,000 food items prepared using United States Department of Agriculture (USDA) publications and also information from food manufacturers. As with any nutritional program, MasterCook calculates the nutritional values of the recipes based on ingredients. Nutrition may vary due to how the food is prepared, where the food comes from, soil content, season, ripeners, processing and methods of preparation. For these reasons, please use the recipes and menu plans as approximate guides. As always, consult your physician and/or a registered dietitian before starting a diet program.

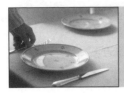

Note: We've included bonus recipes in this study's menu plans. Recipes for *italicized* items in menus can be found in each mealtime section.

🍎 Breakfast

2 low-fat Eggo waffles
½ c. applesauce, sweetened with
1 package artificial sweetener and
2 tbsp. raisins
1 c. nonfat milk
Exchanges: 2 breads, 2 fruits, 1 milk, ½ fat

~~~~~~

1 slice diet whole-wheat bread, toasted
2 tsp. all-fruit spread
1 c. nonfat plain yogurt, artificially sweetened, garnished with
3 tbsp. wheat germ (or 2 tbsp. Grape Nuts)
6 oz. orange juice
Exchanges: 2 breads, 1 fruit, 1 milk

~~~~~~

1 *Banana Muffin*
½ medium cantaloupe
Exchanges: 1 bread, 1 fruit, ½ fat

~~~~~~

1 c. oatmeal with
¼ tsp. reduced-fat margarine
Dash cinnamon
Dash nutmeg
2 tbsp. raisins
1 c. nonfat milk
Exchanges: 1½ breads, 1 fruit, 1 milk, ½ fat

1   *Chewy Fruit-and-Oatmeal Bar*
1   c. sliced strawberries
1   c. nonfat milk

Exchanges: 1 bread, 1 fruit, 1 milk

~~~~~~

1 ½   c. fortified cold cereal
½   small mango
1   c. nonfat milk

Exchanges: 2 breads, 1 fruit, 1 milk

~~~~~~

3   slices diet sourdough bread, toasted
1   tsp. reduced-calorie margarine
¾   c. blueberries
1   c. nonfat milk

Exchanges: 2 breads, 1 fruit, 1 milk, ½ fat

~~~~~~

1   small (2 oz.) bagel
1   tsp. strawberry all-fruit spread
¾   c. artificially sweetened mixed-berry nonfat yogurt
¾   c. blackberries

Exchanges: 2 breads, 1 fruit, 1 milk

~~~~~~

2   low-fat frozen waffles, heated
1   tsp. reduced-calorie margarine
1   tbsp. sugar-free syrup
½   small mango
1   c. nonfat milk

Exchanges: 2 breads, 1/2 fruit, 1 milk, ½ fat

~~~~~~

1   small (2 oz.) whole-wheat English muffin, split and toasted
1   tsp. reduced-calorie margarine
1   c. sliced strawberries
½   c. nonfat milk

Exchanges: 2 breads, 1 fruit, 1 milk, ½ fat

1 c. wheat flakes

1 medium peach, sliced

1 c. nonfat milk

Exchanges: 2 breads, 1 fruit, 1 milk

~~~~~~

1 3-inch canned biscuit, baked

1 tsp. all-fruit spread

½ medium banana

1 c. nonfat milk

Exchanges: 1 bread, 1 fruit, 1 milk, 1 fat

~~~~~~

2 slices diet whole-wheat bread

1 egg, cooked with no added fat

1 strip turkey bacon, cooked crisp

1 medium apple

Exchanges: 1 meat, 1 bread, 1 fruit, ½ fat

~~~~~~

McDonald's Egg McMuffin with no cheese

6 oz. orange juice

Exchanges: 1½ meats, 2 breads, 1 fruit

BONUS BREAKFAST RECIPES

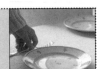

Banana Muffins

1 egg

3 tbsp. vegetable oil

¼ c. nonfat milk

1⅓ c. mashed bananas

1 c. whole-wheat flour

2 tsp. baking powder

¼ tsp. baking soda

⅛ tsp. salt

Nonstick cooking spray

Preheat oven to 400° F. Spray muffin pan with nonstick cooking spray. In large bowl, beat together egg, oil and milk. Stir in bananas and set aside. In separate bowl, combine flour, baking powder, baking soda and salt; mix well. Stir into banana mixture until flour is moistened. Fill each muffin cup ½ to ⅔ full; bake 23 minutes or until tops are lightly browned. Let cool 15 minutes before removing from pans. Serves 12.

Exchanges: ½ bread, ½ fruit, 1 fat

Chewy Fruit-and-Oatmeal Bars

¾ c. brown-sugar substitute

½ c. sugar substitute (not aspartame)

1 8-oz. container plain or vanilla flavored low-fat yogurt

2 egg whites

2 tbsp. applesauce

2 tbsp. nonfat milk

2 tsp. vanilla extract

1½ c. all-purpose flour

1 tsp. baking soda

1 tsp. ground cinnamon

½ tsp. salt

3 c. quick-cooking oats (or old-fashioned oats)

1 c. dried raisins, cranberries or mixed fruit

Preheat oven to 350° F. In large bowl, combine sugar substitutes, yogurt, egg whites, applesauce, milk and vanilla extract; mix well and set aside. In medium bowl, combine flour, baking soda, cinnamon and salt; mix well and blend into yogurt mixture. Stir in oats and dried fruit; spread dough into ungreased 9x13-inch baking dish. Bake 28 to 32 minutes or until light golden brown. Cool completely on wire rack; cut into 24 bars and store in a tightly covered container for up to 2 weeks. Serves 24.

Exchanges: 1 bread

☕ LUNCH

Minestrone Soup

½ can Campbell's Chunky Minestrone soup, heated
8 saltine crackers
1 c. mixed greens with
2 tomato slices and
½ c. baby carrots with
2 tbsp. reduced-fat ranch dressing
½ c. apple juice

Exchanges: 2 breads, 2 vegetables, 1 fat

~~~~~~

Lean Cuisine Lasagna

1 Lean Cuisine Lasagna with Meat Sauce
1 3-inch slice diet French bread, toasted
1 c. spinach, tossed with
½ c. sliced mushrooms and
2 tbsp. reduced-fat French dressing

Exchanges: 2 meats, 2 breads, 1 vegetable, 1 fat

~~~~~~

Chicken Salad

2 c. cooked chicken
1 c. grapes, halved
½ c. finely chopped celery
¼ c. chopped nuts
¼ c. low-fat mayonnaise or Miracle Whip Light
90 low-fat saltine crackers

In a large bowl, combine chicken, grapes, celery, nuts and mayonnaise or Miracle Whip. Spread on crackers. Serves 15.

Exchanges: 1 meat, 1 bread, ½ fat

Healthy Greek Omelet

    3   tbsp. chopped onion
  1 ½   c. torn fresh spinach leaves
    ½   c. Egg Beaters (or other 99% fat-free egg substitute)
    1   oz. feta cheese
        Salt and pepper to taste
        Nonstick cooking spray

In nonstick skillet coated with cooking spray, sauté onions and spinach over medium heat until onions begin to soften and spinach is wilted. Distribute evenly in skillet and cover with egg substitute. When egg begins to set, loosen with spatula and turn over, trying to keep intact. Sprinkle with feta cheese; salt and pepper to taste. Serves 1.

Exchanges: 2 meats, 3 vegetables, 1 fat

~~~~~~

Pita Pizza

    1   6-in. whole-wheat pita
    ¼   c. tomato sauce
        Italian spices (oregano, basil or other seasonings as desired) to taste
        Salt and pepper to taste
    2   oz. part-skim mozzarella cheese
    1   c. sliced portobello mushrooms
    2   small Roma tomatoes, sliced
    1   tsp. grated Romano cheese
    1   tsp. grated Parmesan cheese
        Butter-flavored nonstick cooking spray

Preheat oven to 400° F. Coat pita on both sides with cooking spray; bake 5 minutes or until crispy. Combine tomato sauce with Italian spices, salt and pepper to taste. Spread tomato mixture over pita; layer with mozzarella cheese (reserving about 1 tablespoon), mushrooms and tomatoes. Sprinkle top with Romano and Parmesan cheeses and remaining mozzarella. Garnish with more spices and place back in oven. Baked until cheese is bubbly. Serves 1.

Exchanges: 2 ½ meats, 2 breads, 2 vegetables

Burger King Kid's Meal

　1　small hamburger (without mayonnaise)

　1　small French fries

　1　small diet soda

　1　small apple

Exchanges: 1 ½ meats, 2 ½ breads, 1 fruit, 2 fats

~~~~~~

Superb Chili and Beans

　3　lbs. extra-lean ground beef

　1　lb. pinto beans, rinsed

　1　tbsp. seasoned salt

4 ½　tbsp. chili powder, divided

　2　tsp. cumin, divided

　2　tsp. paprika, divided

　5　qts. plus 2 c. water

　1　c. chopped onion

　1　8-oz. can tomato sauce

　6　garlic cloves, chopped

　1　tsp. oregano

　1　tbsp. salt

　　Salt and pepper to taste

　　Nonstick cooking spray

Combine pinto beans, seasoned salt, 1 tablespoon chili powder, 1 teaspoon cumin, 1 teaspoon paprika and 5 quarts water into 1 ½ -gallon cooking pot. Bring to rolling boil; reduce heat and boil gently 1 ½ hours.

Preheat large nonstick cooking pot coated with cooking spray. Cook beef and onion over medium heat until meat is gray in color; drain excess liquid. Stir in tomato sauce, 2 cups water, 3 ½ tablespoons chili powder, 1 teaspoon cumin, garlic, 1 teaspoon oregano, 1 teaspoon paprika and 1 tablespoon salt. Simmer uncovered 1 hour and 15 minutes.

Meantime, taste pinto beans for seasoning; add salt and pepper, if desired, and continue to gently boil 1 ½ hours more. Add beans to cooked chili and cook 30 minutes more on low heat, stirring often. Serves 20.

Exchanges: 2 meats, 1 bread

Easy Chicken Fajita Wraps

1 oz. boneless, skinless chicken breast, cubed
   Seasoned salt to taste
¼ tsp. garlic powder
1 6-in. whole-wheat tortilla
¼ c. sliced onion
¼ c. sliced green bell pepper
¼ c. shredded lettuce
¼ c. sliced tomato
1 tbsp. low-fat ranch salad dressing

Rub chicken-breast pieces with seasoned salt and garlic powder; let sit 30 minutes.

In small skillet, brown chicken, onion and bell pepper until chicken is cooked through and vegetables are tender-crisp. Arrange chicken mixture onto tortilla; add lettuce, tomato and salad dressing. Fold burrito style and cut in half. Serves 2.

Exchanges: ½ meat, ½ bread, ½ vegetable

~ ~

Chicken with Indian Rice Curry

¾ lb. chicken tenderloins, tendon removed, cut into 1-in. pieces
3 tsp. olive oil
1 small onion, minced
¼ c. chopped tart apple (Braeburn, Granny Smith, Pippin)
   1 to 2 tsp. curry powder
   Dash cayenne pepper
2 c. cooked brown rice
1 c. chickpeas, drained
1 tbsp. fresh lemon juice
½ c. raisins
   Black pepper to taste

Heat large skillet over medium-high heat; then add oil. Sauté chicken pieces 3 minutes or until lightly browned. Add onion; sauté 1 to 2 minutes more. Add apple; sauté additional 1 to 2 minutes. Add curry powder and cayenne pepper to coat mixture; add rice, chickpeas, lemon juice, raisins and black pepper; cook until heated through. Serves 4.

Serve with 1 cup steamed sugar snap peas.

Exchanges: 2 meats, 2 breads, 2 vegetables, 1 fruit, 1 fat

~~~~~~

Taco Bell Lunch

1   Taco Bell Light Chicken Burrito
1   c. gazpacho soup
    small apple

Exchanges: 2 meats, 3 breads, 1 vegetables, 1 fruit

~~~~~~

Pasta Salad

16   oz. penne rigate pasta
 3   qts. water
 4   chicken bouillon cubes
 1   tbsp. seasoned salt
 1   green bell pepper, thinly sliced
 1   red bell pepper, thinly sliced
 1   yellow bell pepper, thinly sliced
 8   oz. mushrooms, thinly sliced
12   black olives, thinly sliced
 1   bunch green onions, tops only, chopped
 1   8-oz. bottle fat-free salad dressing

> **Tip:** To make a meal, top each serving with one of the following:
> - 2 ounces grilled chicken (Add 2 meat exchanges.)
> - 2 ounces shrimp (Add 1 meat exchange.)
> - 2 ounces tuna (Add 1 meat exchange.)

In large saucepan, bring water, bouillon and seasoned salt to boil. Add pasta and boil until tender. Drain liquid; add bell peppers, mushrooms, olives and green onions; toss to mix. Pour dressing over pasta; toss again to coat. Refrigerate until ready to serve. Serves 12.

Exchanges: 2 breads, ½ vegetable

Chicken Noodle Soup Lunch

1 c. prepared canned chicken noodle soup
1 cup broccoli florets with
2 tbsp. fat-free ranch dressing
1 slice Velveeta light cheese
8 low-fat saltines
1 2-in. wedge honeydew melon

Exchanges: 1 meat, 2 breads, 1 vegetable, 1 fruit, 1 fat

~~~~~~

Pearl's Tuna Salad

2 6-oz. cans tuna in water, drained
2 hard-boiled egg whites, diced
½ c. chopped dill pickle
½ c. chopped celery
½ c. chopped green bell pepper
½ c. minced onion
½ c. chopped green onions
2 tbsp. low-fat mayonnaise
1 tbsp. mustard
¼ tsp. seasoned salt
2 tsp. ground black pepper
¼ tsp. cayenne pepper
2 tbsp. parsley
1 tbsp. paprika
1 hard-boiled egg ring for garnish

Combine tuna, egg whites, pickle, celery, bell pepper, onion, green onions, mayonnaise, mustard, seasoned salt, black pepper, cayenne pepper, parsley and paprika in large bowl; mix well. Cover and chill. When ready to serve, garnish with egg ring in the center and sprinkle entire salad with light dusting of paprika. Serves 6.

Exchanges: 1½ meats, ½ vegetable

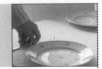

Pinto Beans á la Juan

2	lbs. pinto beans, rinsed
10	qts. water
6	whole garlic cloves
1	large onion, coarsely chopped
1	tbsp. chili powder
1	tbsp. Creole seasoning
1	tbsp. goya adobo
1	tsp. salt

Tip: For added flavor with a cilantro flare, add the following ingredients when beans are tender:

- 2 medium bell peppers, coarsely chopped;
- 4 firm tomatoes, coarsely chopped;
- 1 large yellow onion, coarsely chopped; and
- 1 cilantro bunch, rinsed and tied (discard when done cooking).

(Add $\frac{1}{2}$ vegetable exchange.)

Bring all ingredients to boil in 3-gallon pot. Boil gently 1 $\frac{1}{2}$ hours; taste for seasoning; add more if desired. Continue boiling gently 3 $\frac{1}{2}$ hours more. Serves 24.

Exchanges: 1 bread

~~~~~~

Fat-Free Italian Dressing

1	8-oz. bottle fat-free Italian salad dressing
2	tbsp. balsamic vinegar
1 $\frac{1}{2}$	tbsp. dried basil

Tip: This dressing will last up to 6 months in your refrigerator!

Combine all ingredients in container with lid; shake well to mix thoroughly. Refrigerate until ready to serve.

Exchanges: Free

Aunt Lottie's Crock-Pot Enchiladas

    1   lb. lean ground beef
    1   medium onion, chopped
    1   10.7-oz. can low-fat cream of mushroom soup
    1   10.7-oz. can low-fat cream of chicken soup
    1   16-oz. jar picante sauce
    8   oz. Velveeta Light processed cheese
   12   tortillas, quartered

Brown ground beef and onion in skillet over medium heat. Drain and remove from skillet; set aside. Combine mushroom and chicken soups with picante sauce in small bowl; mix well and set aside. Layer tortillas, browned meat and onions, soup mixture and cheese in Crock-Pot, repeating layers until all ingredients have been used. Cook on high 1 hour or until bubbly. Serves 8.

Exchanges: 3 meats, 1½ breads, 1½ fats

Shepherd's Pie

    1   lb. lean ground beef (or ground sirloin)
    1   small onion, chopped
        Salt and pepper to taste
    1   14.5-oz. can sliced carrots, drained
    1   2-oz. can sliced mushrooms, drained
    4   tbsp. brown gravy mix
    2   c. instant mashed potato flakes
    4   oz. low-fat cheddar cheese

Preheat oven to 350° F. In large skillet over medium-high heat, cook ground beef, onion, salt and pepper until meat is browned. Add carrots and mushrooms; mix gently and reduce heat to simmer. In saucepan, prepare gravy mix according to package directions; slowly stir into meat mixture to distribute evenly. Pour into ungreased 2½-quart baking dish; set aside. Prepare mashed potatoes according to package directions, omitting milk and using only water. Spoon potatoes to form a ring around perimeter of meat; sprinkle cheese over top of potatoes and place in oven just long enough to melt cheese (approximately 3 minutes). Serves 4.

Exchanges: 4 meats, 2 breads, 2 vegetables, ½ milk

~~~~~~

Extraordinary Baked Salmon

  6   4-oz. salmon fillets, each 1 in. thick
  1   tbsp. olive oil
        Splash lemon juice (enough to moisten each fillet)
        Fresh rosemary to taste
        Paprika to taste
        Adobo seasoning to taste
        Black pepper to taste
        Salt to taste
        Honey to taste
  ¼   c. finely chopped pecans
        Nonstick cooking spray

Preheat oven to 450° F. In oven, preheat baking dish drizzled with olive oil. Place fillets skin-side down on flat surface; rub with lemon juice. Sprinkle with seasonings in following order: rosemary, paprika, adobo, black pepper and salt. Lightly drizzle with honey; sprinkle with pecans and seal with generous coating of cooking spray. Place fillets skin-side down in preheated baking dish; bake 10 to 15 minutes or until fillets flake easily with fork. Serves 6.

Exchanges: 3 meats, ½ fat

~~~~~~

Pizza Hut Meal

  2   medium slices Pizza Hut Supreme Thin Crust Pizza
  1   small apple
  2   c. tossed salad with
  2   tbsp. fat-free dressing

Exchanges: 3 meats, 3 breads, 2 vegetables, 1 fruit, 2 fats

Spinach Lasagna

1   10-oz. pkg. frozen chopped spinach, thawed and drained
1   15-oz. pkg. low-fat ricotta cheese
1   c. grated Parmesan cheese, divided
1   c. low-fat plain yogurt
1   egg
¾   tsp. salt
¼   tsp. pepper
1   26-oz. jar low-fat spaghetti sauce
6   lasagna noodles
8   oz. part-skim mozzarella cheese, shredded and divided
1   c. water
    Nonstick cooking spray

Preheat oven to 375° F. Use hands to squeeze out as much excess liquid from spinach as possible. Combine spinach, ricotta cheese, ½ cup Parmesan cheese, yogurt, egg, salt and pepper in large bowl; mix thoroughly and set aside. Evenly spread ½ cup spaghetti sauce in 9x13-inch baking dish coated with cooking spray. Layer 3 lasagna noodles in bottom of dish, breaking last noodle to fit and fill space. Carefully spoon ½ of spinach-cheese mixture to create thin layer over noodles; sprinkle evenly with half of mozzarella cheese. Evenly spread half of remaining spaghetti sauce over cheese and repeat layers beginning with lasagna. Top with remaining Parmesan cheese.

Run a metal spatula or knife around edges of casserole, raising noodles slightly while carefully pouring water around the edges (don't worry if some of the water mixes with the spaghetti sauce). Cover tightly with foil and crimp edges. Bake 1 hour and 15 minutes; remove from oven and let stand covered for 15 minutes. Serves 12.

Exchanges: 1 ½ **meats,** 2 **vegetables,** 1 ½ **fats**

~ ~

Macaroni Casserole

1 Stouffer's Beef Macaroni Casserole
1 c. torn spinach leaves with
  Sliced mushrooms and
1 tbsp. reduced-fat salad dressing
1 peach

Exchanges: 2 meats, 2 breads, 1 vegetable, 1 fruit, 1 fat

~~~~~~

Pork Lo Mein

1 lb. pork tenderloin, cut into thin strips
¼ c. low-sodium soy sauce
3 cloves garlic, minced
1 tsp. minced fresh gingerroot
¼ tsp. cayenne pepper
2 c. snow peas
1 medium red bell pepper, sliced
1 medium yellow bell pepper, sliced
1 medium onion, sliced
3 c. cooked spaghetti
½ c. chicken broth
  Nonstick cooking spray

Combine soy sauce, garlic, gingerroot and cayenne pepper in container;
add pork and marinate 30 minutes. In preheated wok coated with cooking
spray, stir-fry pork together with marinade over high heat 4 to 5 minutes
or until meat is no longer pink. Add snow peas, peppers and onion; stir-fry
until tender. Stir in cooked spaghetti and chicken broth. Cook about 1
minute more or until spaghetti is thoroughly coated. Serves 4.

Exchanges: 3 meats, 1 ½ breads, 2 vegetables

~~~~~~

Ranch-Style Breaded Chicken

4 boneless, skinless chicken breasts
4 oz. fat-free cheddar cheese, shredded
1 1-oz. pkg. ranch dressing mix
20 fat-free saltine crackers, crushed

2 egg whites
Nonstick cooking spray

Preheat oven to 350° F. Place cheese, ranch dressing mix and cracker crumbs each in its own shallow dish or plate; set aside. Slightly beat egg whites in small bowl. One at a time, dip chicken breasts in egg whites; then roll in cheese, dressing mix and cracker crumbs. Place coated chicken breast on baking sheet coated with cooking spray; repeat with remaining breasts. Bake 35 to 40 minutes. Serves 4.

Exchanges: 4 meats, 1 bread

~ ~

Chicken and Pasta Divan

1 Healthy Choice Frozen Chicken and Pasta Divan
Tossed salad with
1 tbsp. reduced-fat dressing
½ c. fruit salad

Exchanges: 2 meats, 2½ breads, 1 vegetable, 1 fruit

~ ~

Grilled Filet Mignon

3 oz. filet mignon, grilled
1 6-ounce baked potato with
1 tsp. margarine
1 tbsp. salsa
1 tbsp. reduced-fat sour cream
½ c. steamed broccoli

Exchanges: 3 meats, 2 breads, 1 vegetable, 1 fat

~ ~

Seafood Restaurant Dinner

1 Broiled or grilled seafood restaurant seafood entrée
(lunch-sized portion, sauce on the side)
½ c. rice
½ c. steamed or grilled vegetables
2 c. salad
2 tbsp. low-fat dressing (on the side)

Exchanges: 3 meats, 2 breads, 2 vegetables, 2 fats

Chili-Chicken Nachos

8	oz. boneless, skinless chicken breasts, cut into thin strips
2	tsp. chili powder
2	tsp. ground cumin
1	tsp. garlic powder
1	tsp. crushed red pepper
1 ½	tsp. fresh oregano
2	10-oz. can tomatoes with green chiles, chunky style
½	c. low-fat cheddar cheese, shredded
4	oz. baked tortilla chips
4	c. shredded lettuce
4	tbsp. fat-free sour cream
1	c. chopped green onions
	Nonstick cooking spray

In large bowl, combine chili powder, cumin, garlic powder, red pepper and oregano; add chicken strips and toss until strips are well coated. Sauté chicken strips in skillet coated with cooking spray using medium heat 7 to 8 minutes or until done. Add tomatoes; simmer 2 to 3 minutes and stir in cheese until melted. Spoon mixture evenly onto 4 plates; top each with 1 ounce tortilla chips, 1 cup lettuce, 1 tablespoon sour cream and ¼ cup chopped green onions. Serves 4.

Exchanges: 2 ½ meats, 1 ½ breads, 1 ½ vegetables, ½ fat

~ ~

Slow-Cooked Orange Chicken

4	3-oz. boneless, skinless chicken breasts
3	c. orange juice
1	c. chopped celery
1	c. chopped green bell pepper
¼	c. chopped onion
½	tsp. salt
¼	tsp. black pepper
3	tbsp. cornstarch
3	tbsp. cold water
1 ⅓	c. cooked rice

Combine chicken, orange juice, celery, bell pepper, onion, salt and pepper in slow cooker; cook on low setting 4 hours or until meat juices run clear.

Combine cornstarch and water until smooth; stir into slow cooker; cover and change setting to high. Cook 30 to 40 minutes. Serve each over ⅓ cup rice. Serves 4.

Exchanges: 3 meats, 1 bread, ½ vegetable, 1 ½ fruits

~~~~~~

Chicken-Stuffed Manicotti

- 2 boneless, skinless chicken breasts
- 12 manicotti pasta shells, cooked and cooled
- 1 c. fat-free sour cream
- 1 10.7-oz. can low-fat cream of chicken soup
- 1 10.7-oz. can low-fat cream of celery soup
- ¼ c. Italian-seasoned bread crumbs
  Nonstick cooking spray

Preheat oven to 350° F. Place chicken in microwave-safe bowl; microwave on high 8 to 10 minutes or until cooked through. Allow to cool; cut into bite-sized pieces. Combine chicken, sour cream, soups and bread crumbs in large bowl; stir well and spoon into manicotti. Arrange filled shells in 7x11-inch baking dish coated with cooking spray; spoon remaining mixture over top. Bake covered 25 minutes. Serves 6.

Exchanges: 1 ½ meats, 2 breads

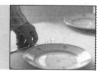

BONUS DINNER RECIPES

Lemon and Basil Carrots

- 1 lb. baby carrots
- 2 tbsp. reduced-calorie margarine
- 1 tbsp. lemon juice
- ½ tsp. garlic powder
- ½ tsp. dried basil
  Dash pepper

Boil carrots in medium saucepan with salted water 20 minutes or until tender; drain and remove from pan. Set aside. In same pan, melt margarine; stir in lemon juice, garlic powder, basil and pepper. Add carrots, cover and toss until carrots are well coated. Let sit 3 minutes before serving. Serves 8.

Exchanges: 1 vegetable, ½ fat

Marinated Italian Green Beans

1   15-oz. can Italian-style green beans, rinsed and drained
½   c. finely chopped onion
¼   c. fat-free Italian dressing

Combine green beans and onion in medium bowl. Add Italian dressing; toss gently to coat. Cover and refrigerate at least 30 minutes. Gently stir again just prior to serving. Serves 4.

Exchanges: 1 vegetable

Pineapple Carrots

1   8-oz. can crushed pineapple in juice,
      drained with 2 tbsp. juice reserved
4   large carrots, julienned
½   c. water
¼   tsp. salt
1   tsp. cornstarch
1   tbsp. snipped parsley
      Salt and pepper to taste

Combine pineapple, water and salt in saucepan. Add carrots; cover and simmer 12 to 15 minutes or until tender. Reduce heat to low. In small bowl or cup, combine reserved pineapple juice and cornstarch, stirring with fork until smooth. Pour mixture slowly into saucepan, stirring constantly. Cook over low heat until bubbly, stirring constantly. Stir in parsley; season to taste with salt and pepper. Serves 4.

Exchanges: ½ vegetable, ½ fruit

☙ SNACKS AND DESSERTS

Apple Cobbler

    6   medium apples, peeled, cored and thinly sliced
    1   6-oz. can frozen apple juice concentrate, unsweetened
        and undiluted
    2   tbsp. cornstarch
    3   tbsp. reduced-fat margarine, divided
    1   tsp. cinnamon
    1   tsp. vanilla extract
    ½   c. flour
    ⅛   tsp. salt
    ⅛   tsp. nutmeg

Preheat oven to 350° F. In a medium saucepan, combine apple juice and cornstarch; cook over medium heat until thick and bubbly. Stir in 1 tablespoon margarine, cinnamon and vanilla extract; add apples and toss to coat. Pour into 9-inch pie plate; set aside. In a separate bowl, mix together flour, salt, nutmeg and 2 tablespoons margarine until crumbly; sprinkle over apple mixture. Bake 30 minutes. Excellent served warm. Serves 8.
Exchanges: 1 ½ fruits, ½ bread, ½ fat

~~~~~~

Creamy Pumpkin Soufflé

    1   1 ½ -oz. box sugar-free vanilla-flavored nonfat instant pudding
    1   c. nonfat milk
    1   16-oz. can pumpkin
    ½   tsp. nutmeg
    ½   tsp. ginger
    ½   tsp. cinnamon
    1   c. fat-free whipped topping

> Tip: Serve as pumpkin pie by pouring the mixture into a reduced-fat graham-cracker piecrust. (Add 1 bread and 1 fat to exchanges.)

Combine pudding mix and milk in medium bowl; stir well. Add pumpkin, nutmeg, ginger and cinnamon; stir. Gently fold in whipped topping; pour into pudding cups. Refrigerate 1 hour or until set. Serves 8.
Exchanges: ½ bread

Light and Luscious Orange Bars

1 envelope plain gelatin

¼ c. frozen orange juice concentrate, thawed

2 tbsp. sugar

½ tsp. vanilla extract

½ c. nonfat powdered milk

½ c. cold water

1 tbsp. lemon juice

24 low-fat graham crackers

Place a small mixing bowl and beaters from electric mixer into refrigerator to chill. Soften gelatin in orange juice concentrate using top section of double boiler, stirring completely over boiling water in bottom section. Remove from heat and stir in sugar and vanilla extract. In chilled bowl, combine powdered milk and cold water; use chilled beaters to beat until soft peaks form. Add lemon juice and beat until stiff; fold in orange juice mixture. Spread evenly on 12 graham crackers; top with remaining graham crackers. Wrap individually in plastic wrap; freeze 2 hours or until firm. Serves 12.

Exchanges: ½ **bread**

Conversion Chart
Equivalent Imperial and Metric Measurements

Liquid Measures

Fluid Ounces	U.S.	Imperial	Milliliters
	1 teaspoon	1 teaspoon	5
$\frac{1}{4}$	2 teaspoons	1 dessert spoon	7
$\frac{1}{2}$	1 tablespoon	1 tablespoon	15
1	2 tablespoons	2 tablespoons	28
2	$\frac{1}{4}$ cup	4 tablespoons	56
4	$\frac{1}{2}$ cup or $\frac{1}{4}$ pint		110
5		$\frac{1}{4}$ pint or 1 gill	140
6	$\frac{3}{4}$ cup		170
8	1 cup or $\frac{1}{2}$ pint		225
9			250 or $\frac{1}{4}$ liter
10	$1\frac{1}{4}$ cups	$\frac{1}{2}$ pint	280
12	$1\frac{1}{2}$ cups or $\frac{3}{4}$ pint		340
15		$\frac{3}{4}$ pint	420
16	2 cups or 1 pint		450
18	$2\frac{1}{4}$ cups		500 or $\frac{1}{2}$ liter
20	$2\frac{1}{2}$ cups	1 pint	560
24	3 cups or $1\frac{1}{2}$ pints		675
25		$1\frac{1}{4}$	700
30	$3\frac{3}{4}$ cups	$1\frac{1}{2}$ pints	840
32	4 cups		900
36	$4\frac{1}{2}$ cups		1,000 or 1 liter
40	5 cups	2 pints or 1 quart	1,120
48	6 cups or 3 pints		1,350
50		$2\frac{1}{2}$ pints	1,400

Solid Measures

U.S. and Imperial Measures		Metric Measures	
Ounces	Pounds	Grams	Kilos
1		28	
2		56	
3½		100	
4	¼	112	
5		140	
6		168	
8	½	225	
9		250	¼
12	¾	340	
16	1	450	
18		500	½
20	1¼	560	
24		675	
27		750	¾
32	2	900	
36	2¼	1,000	1
40	2½	1,100	
48	3	1,350	
54		1,500	1½
64	4	1,800	
72	4½	2,000	2
80	5	2,250	2¼
100	6	2,800	2¾

Oven Temperature Equivalents

Fahrenheit	Celsius	Gas Mark	Description
225	110	$\frac{1}{4}$	Cool
250	130	$\frac{1}{2}$	
275	140	1	Very Slow
300	150	2	
325	170	3	Slow
350	180	4	Moderate
375	190	5	
400	200	6	Moderately Hot
425	220	7	Fairly Hot
450	230	8	Hot
475	240	9	Very Hot
500	250	10	Extremely Hot

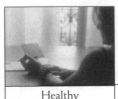

LEADER'S DISCUSSION GUIDE

Healthy
Boundaries

Week One: Acknowledge the Truth

1. **Before the meeting**: Draw three columns on a white board or large piece of butcher paper and label them "Denial," "Delusion" and "Disguise."

2. Recite this week's memory verse as a group.

3. Break into groups of three to four members each. Have each group discuss the correlation between truth and freedom. Have a secretary for each group record the key points in the discussion. After about five minutes, bring the group back together and discuss your findings.

4. Ask for two or three volunteers to tell about a time when acknowledging the truth allowed them to take appropriate action that led to increased freedom.

5. Refer to Day 2. Have the group discuss how the world tells us partial truths about weight loss that distort the truth of God's Word and keep us enslaved to a fad-diet mentality.

6. Ask members to recount how Satan uses the "Deadly Ds" we examined on Day 3 to keep them from achieving success in the First Place program. Write their findings under the appropriate columns you created before the meeting.

7. Have the group discuss some of the paradoxes of the First Place program (e.g., when we spend quiet time with God each morning, we have more time for our other activities; when we eat all of our allotted exchanges, we lose weight).

8. Briefly review the concepts of justification, sanctification and glorification and discuss how each one is part of the Christian life. Be sure to stress the truth of Romans 8:30: Those whom Jesus has justified, He will someday glorify!

9. Ask members to explain how First Place is part of the sanctification process God is using to make them whole and complete.

10. Have members commit to one new behavior they will practice this week that will help them reclaim their heritage as God's children.

11. Close with prayer, thanking Jesus for coming to set us free by allowing us to know the truth.

Week Two: Respond to the Call

1. Last week we looked at the importance of knowing the truth. In order to know the truth, we must first hear the truth. Ask members to identify how denial affects their ability to hear the truth about the condition of their lives.

2. Minimization keeps us from dealing with potentially harmful situations. Ask group members to share how minimizing their health problems keeps them from making a commitment to good health.

3. Have the group discuss how exaggerating the truth keeps a person from getting help. (Paradoxically, many people exaggerate in an attempt to get attention!)

4. On Day 2 we looked at possible reactions to bad news. Go through the choices one by one and have the group talk about why all but one of the choices are self-defeating behaviors.

5. Ask group members what they learned about prayer from studying Nehemiah's example. Have them affirm why going to God in prayer is the only hope of an effective solution.

6. Have group members identify at least one circumstance that God is using in their lives to show the time is right for them to begin rebuilding their damaged boundaries.

7. If God, our King, were to appear to the group today and ask them what they wanted Him to do for them, would their requests keep with God's will for their lives? Ask group members to share three things they would ask God for—things they are confident God would be pleased to give them because they are in harmony with His Word. Keep a master list on a white board or large piece of poster paper. Look for similarities in the group's requests.

8. Discuss the word "response-able" and how First Place teaches us to respond appropriately to God's Word as we care for our bodies.

9. Read 2 Chronicles 20:17 together. Ask members to identify one situation in their lives in which they feel powerless and don't know what to do.

10. Close with prayer. Have each member commit to the Lord the concern he or she shared, confident that Jesus will bring each of you victory.

Week Three: Assess the Damage

1. **Before the meeting**: Write this week's memory verse on a white board or large piece of butcher paper. Under the verse make two columns labeled "Broken City Walls" and "Lack of Self-Control."

2. Discuss correlation between broken walls and lack of self-control. Ask a volunteer to record the group's answers in the two columns you created before the meeting.

3. Ask group members to recall a time when they began boasting about their plans before they carefully planned their course of action, and how making plans public too soon leads to embarrassment.

4. Refer to Day 3. Allow enough time for each group member to share his or her boundary assessment with the group. If your group is larger than 10 members, break the group into smaller groups of three to four members each.

5. Remind group members to encourage one another after each presentation. Don't rush through this exercise; be sure every member has an opportunity to share his or her findings and receive encouragement from the group.

6. Ask the group to share jeers and criticisms they might receive from those who want to discourage their boundary-rebuilding processes. Then have them give appropriate replies to those who may attempt to thwart their plans. Have a volunteer record these comments and replies on a white board or large piece of poster board.

7. Close this week's meeting with a psalm of praise. You can either read Psalm 138 in unison or have members read the words they wrote on Day 7.

Week Four: Reveal False Boundaries

1. **Before the meeting:** Select two or three group members to share their answers to the section of questions in Day 1 in which they substituted their names for David's.

2. Begin by reading all of Psalm 3. You may opt to have eight different group members read one of the eight verses. If you have a small group, you can read the Psalm in unison.

3. Have the volunteers you selected before the meeting share their answers to the section of questions in which they substituted their names for David's.

4. On a whiteboard or a large piece of butcher paper write the word "Idols." Have the group share what they learned about idols from the lesson on Day 2. Have someone in the group record the answers. You may choose to ask a group member to read Isaiah 43:11 to remind the group what God has to say about worshiping idols.

5. Lead a discussion about how false boundaries become idols. If your group is large, you might want to break into smaller groups for this discussion. Try to place at least one mature Christian in each group.

6. Read Paul's words in 1 Corinthians 13:11. Ask members of the group to share childhood thoughts about God that they must demolish so that they can cling to the truth of God's Word. Encourage members to start keeping a list of negative thoughts and the truth of God's Word.

7. Ask members of the group to share how they have used food and/or excess body size as a false boundary so that they would not have to risk abuse or rejection.

8. Lead a discussion about healthy guilt versus compounded guilt. Help members see how guilt can be a false boundary that keeps them from acknowledging a painful truth.

9. Week four contained many painful lessons. Affirm your group for being bold enough to honestly complete the assignments.

10. Close the meeting with a prayer that includes an assurance of pardon.

Week Five: Honor God's Boundaries

1. **Before the meeting**: Write the words "Cost of Commitment" on a whiteboard or large piece of butcher paper.

2. Begin the meeting by reciting Psalm 146 or singing a praise song. Ask members to describe how their spirits are lifted when they praise God.

3. Have the group recite Matthew 6:33 in unison.

4. Briefly review the creation order from the Day 1 lesson (i.e., Creation came about in an orderly fashion and each emerging aspect of creation had everything it needed to thrive before it was created). Ask members to share how studying the creation order assures them that all their needs were met when they put God first in their lives.

5. Discuss how staying within the boundaries of the Live-It plan makes our lives secure. Encourage the group to see the Live-It plan as a God-given boundary that falls in pleasant places.

6. Have someone in the group read 2 Chronicles 20:20-22, and then lead a discussion about how the singers' praise preceded victory.

7. On Day 4 we looked at the connection between obedience and confidence in prayer. Ask members to give a specific example of how they feel more confident when they are within the boundaries of the First Place program on a consistent basis.

8. Ask members to give examples of the cost of discipleship. Select a member to record the group's answers on the white board or piece of paper you prepared before the meeting.

9. End the meeting by having each member pray a one-sentence psalm praise as part of the closing prayer.

Week Six: Take Action Through Prayer

1. **Before the meeting**: Make two columns on a whiteboard or large piece of butcher paper. Label the columns "Crying for Help" and "Responding to the Call."

2. Read Matthew 6:5-8, and then have the group pray the words of the Lord's Prayer (Matthew 6:9-13) in unison.

3. Discuss the two types of prayer (private and corporate) and the place each has in a Christian's prayer life.

4. One of Day 2's assignments was to see how order, humility, praise, obedience and commitment were part of the Lord's Prayer. Have each volunteer take one of the five heart attitudes and share which words of the Lord's Prayer reflect that attitude.

5. Discuss why a willing heart is essential to success in First Place.

6. Read 2 Timothy 2:15 to the group. Ask the group why being able to correctly handle the Word of God is their most important work.

7. Lead a discussion on the responsibilities of the one who calls for help and the one who responds to the call (from Day 5). Ask a volunteer to record the group's answers on the white board or piece of paper you prepared before the meeting.

8. Ask several volunteers to identify a crisis situation in which their spiritual boundaries became blurred and they tried to play God in the life of another human being. Be prepared to first share a personal example. Emphasize that when we lose perspective and forget that God alone saves, we hurt both ourselves and the one we are trying to help.

9   Prayer is not a passive activity. Lead a discussion about how prayer and work are both part of the Christian life.

10. Close by reciting the words of the priestly blessing from Numbers 6:24-26.

Week Seven: Expect Opposition

1. Read 2 Corinthians 2:11, and then lead a discussion on why it is so dangerous to be unaware of Satan's schemes.

2. On Day 1 we identified the real enemy. Have the group discuss how Satan traps people and holds them captive to do his will. Ask the group how that picture changes their perception of the real enemy.

3. Read Genesis 3:1-5, and then lead a discussion about the dangers of trying to dialogue, debate, dispute or dabble in polite conversation with the enemy when he tempts us.

4. Ask members to identify how the Scripture memory commitment of First Place can help them in their struggle against evil.

5. Recite this week's memory verse as a group.

6. Ask three or four members to share how "the sin that so easily entangles" them (Hebrews 12:1) had kept them from obeying the truth.

7. Be sensitive to any in your group who may be victims of domestic violence. Talk about the need to seek help from a pastor or trained counselor and find safety from abuse.

8. Lead a discussion on how busyness often distracts us from obeying the truth.

9. Ask each person to identify one new thing he or she learned this week about the real battle we fight.

10. Emphasize that adhering to the First Place program can give members the needed strength and endurance for their boundary-rebuilding projects. Close with a prayer of recommitment to First Place.

Week Eight: Combat Fatigue and Frustration

1. **Before the meeting**: Look up the words "zeal" and "fervor" in a dictionary. Have these definitions handy during the meeting.

2. Recite this week's memory verse as a group.

3. Lead a discussion about how zeal and fervor apply to the First Place program. These are not everyday words, so use the definitions you gathered to help your group understand what they mean.

4. Ask two of the group members to read their summary on the working conditions described in Nehemiah 4. They could give the report as a TV journalist reports the evening news.

5. Have the group turn to the bar graph they created on Day 2. Go around the room and have each person describe whether their graph was evenly balanced.

6. Have the group discuss the benefits of rest that they discovered on Day 3. If you have a large group, break into groups of three to four members each for this discussion.

7. Living in the moment is a challenge for all of us. Talk about anxiety as it relates to future need, not present want.

8. Read Luke 21:34 to the group. Ask the group to compare the effects of the three conditions Jesus described: dissipation, drunkenness and

anxiety. Once again, if you have a large group, break into smaller groups and then come back together to discuss the findings.

9. Have each person in the group share one thing he or she needs to say no to in order to say yes to First Place wholeheartedly.

10. Role-play ways to tactfully decline invitations and activities that divert us from our First Place goals.

11. Close the meeting with prayer, asking for God's mercy and grace as members grapple with the truths from this week's lesson.

Week Nine: Secure the Heartland

1. **Before the meeting:** Gather a white board or large piece of butcher paper.

2. Recite this week's memory verse as a group.

3. Lead a discussion outlining ways some friends and family members erode our efforts to rebuild healthy lives. As part of your discussion, ask the group how "Reflections" in week seven, Day 6, ties in to the lesson for week nine, Day 1. (You may wish to read the aforementioned "Reflections" to the group.)

4. Have one or more group members read Psalm 139. Discuss the implications of God's knowing, seeing and understanding all we do, and how that affects our integrity.

5. Have separate group members read 2 Chronicles 5:11-14 and Philippians 4:4-5, and then lead a discussion on the connection between praise and protection.

6. Read the Nine Commitments one by one while brainstorming how each is a limitation that protects us.

7. On a whiteboard or large piece of butcher paper, list positive ways to deal with emotions and thoughts that could potentially harm ourselves or others if not handled correctly.

8. End the lesson with a praise song. Ask a musically gifted member of your group to help you find a song that speaks of God's faithful protection of His children.

Week Ten: Reclaim God's Promises

1. **Before the meeting**: Make two columns on a white board or large piece of butcher paper. Label the columns "Self-Serving Freedom" and "Freedom to Worship God." Adjacent to that list or on another piece of paper, write the words "Hearing," "Praising," "Weeping," "Rejoicing" and "Sharing."

2. Read the account of the transfiguration in Mark 9:2-10 to the group as a background for this week's memory verse.

3. Lead a discussion on why listening is so important to a right relationship with God.

4. Ask the group to give examples of self-serving freedom and freedom to worship God as they relate to the First Place program. Have a volunteer write the group's answers on the white board or piece of paper you prepared before the meeting.

5. Discuss the importance of having ears to hear what the Spirit says.

6. Have the group give examples of how hearing, praising, weeping, rejoicing and sharing are forms of worshiping God. Record their findings on the second list you prepared before the meeting.

7. Choose a member to read the parable of the wise and foolish builders found in Matthew 7:24-27. Lead a discussion on what differentiates the wise from the foolish. Emphasize that Jesus did not say if the storm were to come; He said when the storm came. Tribulation is certain. How we handle tribulation depends on our foundation.

8. Go around the room and ask each person to name two things he or she learned from this Bible study and how these lessons will help him or her succeed in First Place.

9. Lead a prayer of confession followed by a time of praise.

PERSONAL WEIGHT RECORD

Week	Weight	+ or -	Goal This Session	Pounds to Goal
1				
2				
3				
4				
5				
6				
7				
8				
9				
10				
11				
12				
13				
Final				

Beginning Measurements

Waist_____ Hips_____ Thighs_____ Chest_____

Ending Measurements

Waist_____ Hips_____ Thighs_____ Chest_____

COMMITMENT RECORDS

How to Fill Out a Commitment Record

The Commitment Record (CR) is an aid for you in keeping track of your accomplishments. Begin a new CR on the morning of the day your class meets. This ensures that your CR is complete before your next meeting. Turn in the CR weekly to your leader.

FIRST PLACE CR

Name_____

Date_____through _____

Week # _____ Calorie Level _____ → Choose your calorie level.

Daily Exchange Plan

Level	Meat	Bread	Veggie	Fruit	Milk	Fat
1200	4-5	5-6	3	2-3	2-3	3-4
1400	5-6	6-7	3-4	3-4	2-3	3-4
1500	5-6	7-8	3-4	3-4	2-3	3-4
1600	6-7	8-9	3-4	3-4	2-3	3-4
1800	6-7	10-11	3-4	3-4	2-3	4-5
2000	6-7	11-12	4-5	4-5	2-3	4-5
2200	7-8	12-13	4-5	4-5	2-3	6-7
2400	8-9	13-14	4-5	4-5	2-3	7-8
2600	9-10	14-15	5	5	2-3	7-8
2800	9-10	15-16	5	5	2-3	9

Limit your high-range selections to only one of the following each day: meat, bread, milk or fat.

Weekly Progress

_____Loss _____Gain _____Maintain

___ Attendance ___ Bible Study
___ Prayer ___ Scripture Reading
___ Memory Verse ___ CR
___ Encouragement _____
___ Exercise:

Aerobic _____

_____

Strength _____

Flexibility _____

At the end of each week, complete the weekly progress.

Record the number of days you kept the commitment.

Write the initials of the group member you encouraged this week.

DAY 7: Date _____

Morning _____

_____

Midday _____

_____

Evening _____

_____

Snacks _____

_____

___ Meet _____   ☐ Prayer
___ Bread _____   ☐ Bible Study
___ Vegetable ____   ☐ Scripture Reading
___ Fruit _____   ☐ Memory Verse
___ Milk _____   ☐ Encouragement
___ Fat _____   ☐ Water_____

Exercise

Aerobic _____

_____

Strength _____

Flexibility _____

List the foods you have eaten. On this condensed CR it is not necessary to exchange each food choice. It will be the responsibility of each member that the tally marks you list below are accurate regarding each food choice. If you are unsure of an exchange, check the Live-It section of your copy of the *Member's Guide*.

List the daily food exchange choices to the left of the food groups.

Use tally marks for the actual food and water consumed.

Check off commitments completed. Use tally marks to record each 8-oz. serving of water.

List type and duration of exercise.

FIRST PLACE CR

Name _____

Date _____ through _____

Week # _____ Calorie Level _____

Daily Exchange Plan

Level	Meat	Bread	Veggie	Fruit	Milk	Fat
1200	4-5	5-6	3	2-3	2-3	3-4
1400	5-6	6-7	3-4	3-4	2-3	3-4
1500	5-6	7-8	3-4	3-4	2-3	3-4
1600	6-7	8-9	3-4	3-4	2-3	3-4
1800	6-7	10-11	3-4	3-4	2-3	4-5
2000	6-7	11-12	4-5	4-5	2-3	4-5
2200	7-8	12-13	4-5	4-5	2-3	6-7
2400	8-9	13-14	4-5	4-5	2-3	7-8
2600	9-10	14-15	5	5	2-3	7-8
2800	9-10	15-16	5	5	2-3	9

You may always choose the high range of vegetables and fruits. Limit your high range selections to only one of the following: meat, bread, milk or fat.

Weekly Progress

____ Loss ____ Gain ____ Maintain

____ Attendance ____ Bible Study
____ Prayer ____ Scripture Reading
____ Memory Verse ____ CR
____ Encouragement:
____ Exercise
Aerobic _____

Strength _____
Flexibility _____

DAY 5: Date _____

Morning _____
_____

Midday _____
_____
_____

Evening _____
_____
_____

Snacks _____
_____

____ Meat   ☐ Prayer
____ Bread   ☐ Bible Study
____ Vegetable   ☐ Scripture Reading
____ Fruit   ☐ Memory Verse
____ Milk   ☐ Encouragement
____ Fat   ☐ Water

Exercise
Aerobic _____

Strength _____
Flexibility _____

DAY 6: Date _____

Morning _____
_____

Midday _____
_____
_____

Evening _____
_____
_____

Snacks _____
_____

____ Meat   ☐ Prayer
____ Bread   ☐ Bible Study
____ Vegetable   ☐ Scripture Reading
____ Fruit   ☐ Memory Verse
____ Milk   ☐ Encouragement
____ Fat   ☐ Water

Exercise
Aerobic _____

Strength _____
Flexibility _____

DAY 7: Date _____

Morning _____
_____

Midday _____
_____
_____

Evening _____
_____
_____

Snacks _____
_____

____ Meat   ☐ Prayer
____ Bread   ☐ Bible Study
____ Vegetable   ☐ Scripture Reading
____ Fruit   ☐ Memory Verse
____ Milk   ☐ Encouragement
____ Fat   ☐ Water

Exercise
Aerobic _____

Strength _____
Flexibility _____

DAY 1: Date _____

Morning _____

Midday _____

Evening _____

Snacks _____

___ Meat	☐ Prayer
___ Bread	☐ Bible Study
___ Vegetable	☐ Scripture Reading
___ Fruit	☐ Memory Verse
___ Milk	☐ Encouragement
___ Fat	___ Water

Exercise
Aerobic _____
Strength _____
Flexibility _____

DAY 2: Date _____

Morning _____

Midday _____

Evening _____

Snacks _____

___ Meat	☐ Prayer
___ Bread	☐ Bible Study
___ Vegetable	☐ Scripture Reading
___ Fruit	☐ Memory Verse
___ Milk	☐ Encouragement
___ Fat	___ Water

Exercise
Aerobic _____
Strength _____
Flexibility _____

DAY 3: Date _____

Morning _____

Midday _____

Evening _____

Snacks _____

___ Meat	☐ Prayer
___ Bread	☐ Bible Study
___ Vegetable	☐ Scripture Reading
___ Fruit	☐ Memory Verse
___ Milk	☐ Encouragement
___ Fat	___ Water

Exercise
Aerobic _____
Strength _____
Flexibility _____

DAY 4: Date _____

Morning _____

Midday _____

Evening _____

Snacks _____

___ Meat	☐ Prayer
___ Bread	☐ Bible Study
___ Vegetable	☐ Scripture Reading
___ Fruit	☐ Memory Verse
___ Milk	☐ Encouragement
___ Fat	___ Water

Exercise
Aerobic _____
Strength _____
Flexibility _____

FIRST PLACE CR

DAY 5: Date _____ DAY 6: Date _____ DAY 7: Date _____

Name _____
Date _____ through _____
Week # ____ Calorie Level _____

Daily Exchange Plan

Level	Meat	Bread	Veggie	Fruit	Milk	Fat
1200	4-5	5-6	3	2-3	2-3	3-4
1400	5-6	6-7	3-4	3-4	2-3	3-4
1500	5-6	7-8	3-4	3-4	2-3	3-4
1600	6-7	8-9	3-4	3-4	2-3	3-4
1800	6-7	10-11	3-4	3-4	2-3	4-5
2000	6-7	11-12	4-5	4-5	2-3	4-5
2200	7-8	12-13	4-5	4-5	2-3	6-7
2400	8-9	13-14	4-5	4-5	2-3	7-8
2600	9-10	14-15	5	5	2-3	7-8
2800	9-10	15-16	5	5	2-3	9

You may always choose the high range of vegetables and fruits. Limit your high range selections to only one of the following: meat, bread, milk or fat.

Weekly Progress

____ Loss ____ Gain ____ Maintain

____ Attendance ____ Bible Study
____ Prayer ____ Scripture Reading
____ Memory Verse ____ CR
____ Encouragement:
____ Exercise
Aerobic _____
Strength _____
Flexibility _____

DAY 7:

Morning _____
Midday _____
Evening _____
Snacks _____

____ Meat ☐ Prayer
____ Bread ☐ Bible Study
____ Vegetable ☐ Scripture Reading
____ Fruit ☐ Memory Verse
____ Milk ☐ Encouragement
____ Fat ☐ Water
Exercise
Aerobic _____
Strength _____
Flexibility _____

DAY 6:

Morning _____
Midday _____
Evening _____
Snacks _____

____ Meat ☐ Prayer
____ Bread ☐ Bible Study
____ Vegetable ☐ Scripture Reading
____ Fruit ☐ Memory Verse
____ Milk ☐ Encouragement
____ Fat ☐ Water
Exercise
Aerobic _____
Strength _____
Flexibility _____

DAY 5:

Morning _____
Midday _____
Evening _____
Snacks _____

____ Meat ☐ Prayer
____ Bread ☐ Bible Study
____ Vegetable ☐ Scripture Reading
____ Fruit ☐ Memory Verse
____ Milk ☐ Encouragement
____ Fat ☐ Water
Exercise
Aerobic _____
Strength _____
Flexibility _____

DAY 1: Date _____

Morning _____

Midday _____

Evening _____

Snacks _____

___ Meat	☐ Prayer
___ Bread	☐ Bible Study
___ Vegetable	☐ Scripture Reading
___ Fruit	☐ Memory Verse
___ Milk	☐ Encouragement
___ Fat ___ Water	

Exercise
Aerobic _____
Strength _____
Flexibility _____

DAY 2: Date _____

Morning _____

Midday _____

Evening _____

Snacks _____

___ Meat	☐ Prayer
___ Bread	☐ Bible Study
___ Vegetable	☐ Scripture Reading
___ Fruit	☐ Memory Verse
___ Milk	☐ Encouragement
___ Fat ___ Water	

Exercise
Aerobic _____
Strength _____
Flexibility _____

DAY 3: Date _____

Morning _____

Midday _____

Evening _____

Snacks _____

___ Meat	☐ Prayer
___ Bread	☐ Bible Study
___ Vegetable	☐ Scripture Reading
___ Fruit	☐ Memory Verse
___ Milk	☐ Encouragement
___ Fat ___ Water	

Exercise
Aerobic _____
Strength _____
Flexibility _____

DAY 4: Date _____

Morning _____

Midday _____

Evening _____

Snacks _____

___ Meat	☐ Prayer
___ Bread	☐ Bible Study
___ Vegetable	☐ Scripture Reading
___ Fruit	☐ Memory Verse
___ Milk	☐ Encouragement
___ Fat ___ Water	

Exercise
Aerobic _____
Strength _____
Flexibility _____

FIRST PLACE CR

Name _____

Date _____ through _____

Week # _____ Calorie Level _____

Daily Exchange Plan

Level	Meat	Bread	Veggie	Fruit	Milk	Fat
1200	4-5	5-6	3	2-3	2-3	3-4
1400	5-6	6-7	3-4	3-4	2-3	3-4
1500	5-6	7-8	3-4	3-4	2-3	3-4
1600	6-7	8-9	3-4	3-4	2-3	3-4
1800	6-7	10-11	3-4	3-4	2-3	4-5
2000	6-7	11-12	4-5	4-5	2-3	4-5
2200	7-8	12-13	4-5	4-5	2-3	6-7
2400	8-9	13-14	4-5	4-5	2-3	7-8
2600	9-10	14-15	5	5	2-3	7-8
2800	9-10	15-16	5	5	2-3	9

You may always choose the high range of vegetables and fruits. Limit your high range selections to only one of the following: meat, bread, milk or fat.

Weekly Progress

_____ Loss _____ Gain _____ Maintain

_____ Attendance _____ Bible Study
_____ Prayer _____ Scripture Reading
_____ Memory Verse _____ CR
_____ Encouragement:
_____ Exercise

Aerobic _____

Strength _____
Flexibility _____

DAY 5: Date _____

Morning _____

Midday _____

Evening _____

Snacks _____

_____ Meat   ☐ Prayer
_____ Bread   ☐ Bible Study
_____ Vegetable   ☐ Scripture Reading
_____ Fruit   ☐ Memory Verse
_____ Milk   ☐ Encouragement
_____ Fat   Water _____

Exercise
Aerobic _____

Strength _____
Flexibility _____

DAY 6: Date _____

Morning _____

Midday _____

Evening _____

Snacks _____

_____ Meat   ☐ Prayer
_____ Bread   ☐ Bible Study
_____ Vegetable   ☐ Scripture Reading
_____ Fruit   ☐ Memory Verse
_____ Milk   ☐ Encouragement
_____ Fat   Water _____

Exercise
Aerobic _____

Strength _____
Flexibility _____

DAY 7: Date _____

Morning _____

Midday _____

Evening _____

Snacks _____

_____ Meat   ☐ Prayer
_____ Bread   ☐ Bible Study
_____ Vegetable   ☐ Scripture Reading
_____ Fruit   ☐ Memory Verse
_____ Milk   ☐ Encouragement
_____ Fat   Water _____

Exercise
Aerobic _____

Strength _____
Flexibility _____

DAY 1: Date _____

Morning _____

Midday _____

Evening _____

Snacks _____

___ Meat	☐ Prayer
___ Bread	☐ Bible Study
___ Vegetable	☐ Scripture Reading
___ Fruit	☐ Memory Verse
___ Milk	☐ Encouragement
___ Fat	___ Water

Exercise
Aerobic _____
Strength _____
Flexibility _____

DAY 2: Date _____

Morning _____

Midday _____

Evening _____

Snacks _____

___ Meat	☐ Prayer
___ Bread	☐ Bible Study
___ Vegetable	☐ Scripture Reading
___ Fruit	☐ Memory Verse
___ Milk	☐ Encouragement
___ Fat	___ Water

Exercise
Aerobic _____
Strength _____
Flexibility _____

DAY 3: Date _____

Morning _____

Midday _____

Evening _____

Snacks _____

___ Meat	☐ Prayer
___ Bread	☐ Bible Study
___ Vegetable	☐ Scripture Reading
___ Fruit	☐ Memory Verse
___ Milk	☐ Encouragement
___ Fat	___ Water

Exercise
Aerobic _____
Strength _____
Flexibility _____

DAY 4: Date _____

Morning _____

Midday _____

Evening _____

Snacks _____

___ Meat	☐ Prayer
___ Bread	☐ Bible Study
___ Vegetable	☐ Scripture Reading
___ Fruit	☐ Memory Verse
___ Milk	☐ Encouragement
___ Fat	___ Water

Exercise
Aerobic _____
Strength _____
Flexibility _____

FIRST PLACE CR

Name _____

Date _____ through _____

Week # _____ Calorie Level _____

Daily Exchange Plan

Level	Meat	Bread	Veggie	Fruit	Milk	Fat
1200	4-5	5-6	3	2-3	2-3	3-4
1400	5-6	6-7	3-4	3-4	2-3	3-4
1500	5-6	7-8	3-4	3-4	2-3	3-4
1600	6-7	8-9	3-4	3-4	2-3	3-4
1800	6-7	10-11	3-4	3-4	2-3	4-5
2000	6-7	11-12	4-5	4-5	2-3	4-5
2200	7-8	12-13	4-5	4-5	2-3	6-7
2400	8-9	13-14	4-5	4-5	2-3	7-8
2600	9-10	14-15	5	5	2-3	7-8
2800	9-10	15-16	5	5	2-3	9

You may always choose the high range of vegetables and fruits. Limit your high range selections to only one of the following: meat, bread, milk or fat.

Weekly Progress

_____ Loss _____ Gain _____ Maintain

_____ Attendance _____ Bible Study
_____ Prayer _____ Scripture Reading
_____ Memory Verse _____ CR
_____ Encouragement:
_____ Exercise
Aerobic _____
Strength _____
Flexibility _____

DAY 5: Date _____

Morning _____

Midday _____

Evening _____

Snacks _____

_____ Meat   □ Prayer
_____ Bread   □ Bible Study
_____ Vegetable □ Scripture Reading
_____ Fruit   □ Memory Verse
_____ Milk   □ Encouragement
_____ Fat   Water _____

Exercise
Aerobic _____

Strength _____
Flexibility _____

DAY 6: Date _____

Morning _____

Midday _____

Evening _____

Snacks _____

_____ Meat   □ Prayer
_____ Bread   □ Bible Study
_____ Vegetable □ Scripture Reading
_____ Fruit   □ Memory Verse
_____ Milk   □ Encouragement
_____ Fat   Water _____

Exercise
Aerobic _____

Strength _____
Flexibility _____

DAY 7: Date _____

Morning _____

Midday _____

Evening _____

Snacks _____

_____ Meat   □ Prayer
_____ Bread   □ Bible Study
_____ Vegetable □ Scripture Reading
_____ Fruit   □ Memory Verse
_____ Milk   □ Encouragement
_____ Fat   Water _____

Exercise
Aerobic _____

Strength _____
Flexibility _____

DAY 1: Date _____

Morning _____

Midday _____

Evening _____

Snacks _____

Meat _____	☐ Prayer
Bread _____	☐ Bible Study
Vegetable _____	☐ Scripture Reading
Fruit _____	☐ Memory Verse
Milk _____	☐ Encouragement
Fat _____	Water _____

Exercise
Aerobic _____
Strength _____
Flexibility _____

DAY 2: Date _____

Morning _____

Midday _____

Evening _____

Snacks _____

Meat _____	☐ Prayer
Bread _____	☐ Bible Study
Vegetable _____	☐ Scripture Reading
Fruit _____	☐ Memory Verse
Milk _____	☐ Encouragement
Fat _____	Water _____

Exercise
Aerobic _____
Strength _____
Flexibility _____

DAY 3: Date _____

Morning _____

Midday _____

Evening _____

Snacks _____

Meat _____	☐ Prayer
Bread _____	☐ Bible Study
Vegetable _____	☐ Scripture Reading
Fruit _____	☐ Memory Verse
Milk _____	☐ Encouragement
Fat _____	Water _____

Exercise
Aerobic _____
Strength _____
Flexibility _____

DAY 4: Date _____

Morning _____

Midday _____

Evening _____

Snacks _____

Meat _____	☐ Prayer
Bread _____	☐ Bible Study
Vegetable _____	☐ Scripture Reading
Fruit _____	☐ Memory Verse
Milk _____	☐ Encouragement
Fat _____	Water _____

Exercise
Aerobic _____
Strength _____
Flexibility _____

FIRST PLACE CR

Name _____

Date _____ through _____

Week # _____ Calorie Level _____

Daily Exchange Plan

Level	Meat	Bread	Veggie	Fruit	Milk	Fat
1200	4-5	5-6	3	2-3	2-3	3-4
1400	5-6	6-7	3-4	3-4	2-3	3-4
1500	5-6	7-8	3-4	3-4	2-3	3-4
1600	6-7	8-9	3-4	3-4	2-3	3-4
1800	6-7	10-11	3-4	3-4	2-3	4-5
2000	6-7	11-12	4-5	4-5	2-3	4-5
2200	7-8	12-13	4-5	4-5	2-3	6-7
2400	8-9	13-14	4-5	4-5	2-3	7-8
2600	9-10	14-15	5	5	2-3	7-8
2800	9-10	15-16	5	5	2-3	9

You may always choose the high range of vegetables and fruits. Limit your high range selections to only one of the following: meat, bread, milk or fat.

Weekly Progress

____ Loss   ____ Gain   ____ Maintain

____ Attendance   ____ Bible Study
____ Prayer   ____ Scripture Reading
____ Memory Verse   ____ CR
____ Encouragement:
____ Exercise
Aerobic _____
Strength _____
Flexibility _____

DAY 5: Date _____

Morning _____

Midday _____

Evening _____

Snacks _____
_____

____ Meat   ☐ Prayer
____ Bread   ☐ Bible Study
____ Vegetable   ☐ Scripture Reading
____ Fruit   ☐ Memory Verse
____ Milk   ☐ Encouragement
____ Fat   ____ Water

Exercise
Aerobic _____

Strength _____
Flexibility _____

DAY 6: Date _____

Morning _____

Midday _____

Evening _____

Snacks _____
_____

____ Meat   ☐ Prayer
____ Bread   ☐ Bible Study
____ Vegetable   ☐ Scripture Reading
____ Fruit   ☐ Memory Verse
____ Milk   ☐ Encouragement
____ Fat   ____ Water

Exercise
Aerobic _____

Strength _____
Flexibility _____

DAY 7: Date _____

Morning _____

Midday _____

Evening _____

Snacks _____
_____

____ Meat   ☐ Prayer
____ Bread   ☐ Bible Study
____ Vegetable   ☐ Scripture Reading
____ Fruit   ☐ Memory Verse
____ Milk   ☐ Encouragement
____ Fat   ____ Water

Exercise
Aerobic _____

Strength _____
Flexibility _____

DAY 1: Date _____

Morning _____

Midday _____

Evening _____

Snacks _____

Meat _____	☐ Prayer
Bread _____	☐ Bible Study
Vegetable _____	☐ Scripture Reading
Fruit _____	☐ Memory Verse
Milk _____	☐ Encouragement
Fat _____	Water _____

Exercise
Aerobic _____
Strength _____
Flexibility _____

DAY 2: Date _____

Morning _____

Midday _____

Evening _____

Snacks _____

Meat _____	☐ Prayer
Bread _____	☐ Bible Study
Vegetable _____	☐ Scripture Reading
Fruit _____	☐ Memory Verse
Milk _____	☐ Encouragement
Fat _____	Water _____

Exercise
Aerobic _____
Strength _____
Flexibility _____

DAY 3: Date _____

Morning _____

Midday _____

Evening _____

Snacks _____

Meat _____	☐ Prayer
Bread _____	☐ Bible Study
Vegetable _____	☐ Scripture Reading
Fruit _____	☐ Memory Verse
Milk _____	☐ Encouragement
Fat _____	Water _____

Exercise
Aerobic _____
Strength _____
Flexibility _____

DAY 4: Date _____

Morning _____

Midday _____

Evening _____

Snacks _____

Meat _____	☐ Prayer
Bread _____	☐ Bible Study
Vegetable _____	☐ Scripture Reading
Fruit _____	☐ Memory Verse
Milk _____	☐ Encouragement
Fat _____	Water _____

Exercise
Aerobic _____
Strength _____
Flexibility _____

FIRST PLACE CR

Name _____

Date _____ through _____

Week # _____ Calorie Level _____

Daily Exchange Plan

Level	Meat	Bread	Veggie	Fruit	Milk	Fat
1200	4-5	5-6	3	2-3	2-3	3-4
1400	5-6	6-7	3-4	3-4	2-3	3-4
1500	5-6	7-8	3-4	3-4	2-3	3-4
1600	6-7	8-9	3-4	3-4	2-3	3-4
1800	6-7	10-11	3-4	3-4	2-3	4-5
2000	6-7	11-12	4-5	4-5	2-3	4-5
2200	7-8	12-13	4-5	4-5	2-3	6-7
2400	8-9	13-14	4-5	4-5	2-3	7-8
2600	9-10	14-15	5	5	2-3	7-8
2800	9-10	15-16	5	5	2-3	9

You may always choose the high range of vegetables and fruits. Limit your high range selections to only one of the following: meat, bread, milk or fat.

Weekly Progress

_____ Loss _____ Gain _____ Maintain

_____ Attendance _____ Bible Study

_____ Prayer _____ Scripture Reading

_____ Memory Verse _____ CR

_____ Encouragement: _____

_____ Exercise _____

Aerobic _____

Strength _____

Flexibility _____

DAY 5: Date _____

Morning _____

_____

Midday _____

_____

Evening _____

_____

Snacks _____

_____

_____ Meat   ☐ Prayer

_____ Bread   ☐ Bible Study

_____ Vegetable   ☐ Scripture Reading

_____ Fruit   ☐ Memory Verse

_____ Milk   ☐ Encouragement

_____ Fat   Water _____

Exercise

Aerobic _____

Strength _____

Flexibility _____

DAY 6: Date _____

Morning _____

_____

Midday _____

_____

Evening _____

_____

Snacks _____

_____

_____ Meat   ☐ Prayer

_____ Bread   ☐ Bible Study

_____ Vegetable   ☐ Scripture Reading

_____ Fruit   ☐ Memory Verse

_____ Milk   ☐ Encouragement

_____ Fat   Water _____

Exercise

Aerobic _____

Strength _____

Flexibility _____

DAY 7: Date _____

Morning _____

_____

Midday _____

_____

Evening _____

_____

Snacks _____

_____

_____ Meat   ☐ Prayer

_____ Bread   ☐ Bible Study

_____ Vegetable   ☐ Scripture Reading

_____ Fruit   ☐ Memory Verse

_____ Milk   ☐ Encouragement

_____ Fat   Water _____

Exercise

Aerobic _____

Strength _____

Flexibility _____

DAY 1: Date _____

Morning _____

Midday _____

Evening _____

Snacks _____

___ Meat	☐ Prayer
___ Bread	☐ Bible Study
___ Vegetable	☐ Scripture Reading
___ Fruit	☐ Memory Verse
___ Milk	☐ Encouragement
___ Fat	___ Water

Exercise

Aerobic _____

Strength _____

Flexibility _____

DAY 2: Date _____

Morning _____

Midday _____

Evening _____

Snacks _____

___ Meat	☐ Prayer
___ Bread	☐ Bible Study
___ Vegetable	☐ Scripture Reading
___ Fruit	☐ Memory Verse
___ Milk	☐ Encouragement
___ Fat	___ Water

Exercise

Aerobic _____

Strength _____

Flexibility _____

DAY 3: Date _____

Morning _____

Midday _____

Evening _____

Snacks _____

___ Meat	☐ Prayer
___ Bread	☐ Bible Study
___ Vegetable	☐ Scripture Reading
___ Fruit	☐ Memory Verse
___ Milk	☐ Encouragement
___ Fat	___ Water

Exercise

Aerobic _____

Strength _____

Flexibility _____

DAY 4: Date _____

Morning _____

Midday _____

Evening _____

Snacks _____

___ Meat	☐ Prayer
___ Bread	☐ Bible Study
___ Vegetable	☐ Scripture Reading
___ Fruit	☐ Memory Verse
___ Milk	☐ Encouragement
___ Fat	___ Water

Exercise

Aerobic _____

Strength _____

Flexibility _____

FIRST PLACE CR

Name _____

Date _____ through _____

Week # _____   Calorie Level _____

Daily Exchange Plan

Level	Meat	Bread	Veggie	Fruit	Milk	Fat
1200	4-5	5-6	3	2-3	2-3	3-4
1400	5-6	6-7	3-4	3-4	2-3	3-4
1500	5-6	7-8	3-4	3-4	2-3	3-4
1600	6-7	8-9	3-4	3-4	2-3	3-4
1800	6-7	10-11	3-4	3-4	2-3	4-5
2000	6-7	11-12	4-5	4-5	2-3	4-5
2200	7-8	12-13	4-5	4-5	2-3	6-7
2400	8-9	13-14	4-5	4-5	2-3	7-8
2600	9-10	14-15	5	5	2-3	7-8
2800	9-10	15-16	5	5	2-3	9

You may always choose the high range of vegetables and fruits. Limit your high range selections to only one of the following: meat, bread, milk or fat.

Weekly Progress

_____ Loss   _____ Gain   _____ Maintain

_____ Attendance   _____ Bible Study
_____ Prayer   _____ Scripture Reading
_____ Memory Verse   _____ CR
_____ Encouragement:
_____ Exercise
       Aerobic

Strength _____
Flexibility _____

DAY 5: Date _____

Morning _____

Midday _____

Evening _____

Snacks _____

_____ Meat
_____ Bread
_____ Vegetable
_____ Fruit
_____ Milk
_____ Fat
Exercise
Aerobic _____

☐ Prayer
☐ Bible Study
☐ Scripture Reading
☐ Memory Verse
☐ Encouragement
_____ Water

Strength _____
Flexibility _____

DAY 6: Date _____

Morning _____

Midday _____

Evening _____

Snacks _____

_____ Meat
_____ Bread
_____ Vegetable
_____ Fruit
_____ Milk
_____ Fat
Exercise
Aerobic _____

☐ Prayer
☐ Bible Study
☐ Scripture Reading
☐ Memory Verse
☐ Encouragement
_____ Water

Strength _____
Flexibility _____

DAY 7: Date _____

Morning _____

Midday _____

Evening _____

Snacks _____

_____ Meat
_____ Bread
_____ Vegetable
_____ Fruit
_____ Milk
_____ Fat
Exercise
Aerobic _____

☐ Prayer
☐ Bible Study
☐ Scripture Reading
☐ Memory Verse
☐ Encouragement
_____ Water

Strength _____
Flexibility _____

DAY 1: Date _____

Morning _____

Midday _____

Evening _____

Snacks _____

____ Meat   ☐ Prayer
____ Bread   ☐ Bible Study
____ Vegetable   ☐ Scripture Reading
____ Fruit   ☐ Memory Verse
____ Milk   ☐ Encouragement
____ Fat   ____ Water

Exercise
Aerobic _____
Strength _____
Flexibility _____

DAY 2: Date _____

Morning _____

Midday _____

Evening _____

Snacks _____

____ Meat   ☐ Prayer
____ Bread   ☐ Bible Study
____ Vegetable   ☐ Scripture Reading
____ Fruit   ☐ Memory Verse
____ Milk   ☐ Encouragement
____ Fat   ____ Water

Exercise
Aerobic _____
Strength _____
Flexibility _____

DAY 3: Date _____

Morning _____

Midday _____

Evening _____

Snacks _____

____ Meat   ☐ Prayer
____ Bread   ☐ Bible Study
____ Vegetable   ☐ Scripture Reading
____ Fruit   ☐ Memory Verse
____ Milk   ☐ Encouragement
____ Fat   ____ Water

Exercise
Aerobic _____
Strength _____
Flexibility _____

DAY 4: Date _____

Morning _____

Midday _____

Evening _____

Snacks _____

____ Meat   ☐ Prayer
____ Bread   ☐ Bible Study
____ Vegetable   ☐ Scripture Reading
____ Fruit   ☐ Memory Verse
____ Milk   ☐ Encouragement
____ Fat   ____ Water

Exercise
Aerobic _____
Strength _____
Flexibility _____

FIRST PLACE CR

Name _____

Date _____ through _____

Week # _____ Calorie Level _____

Daily Exchange Plan

Level	Meat	Bread	Veggie	Fruit	Milk	Fat
1200	4-5	5-6	3	2-3	2-3	3-4
1400	5-5	6-7	3-4	3-4	2-3	3-4
1500	5-5	7-8	3-4	3-4	2-3	3-4
1600	6-7	8-9	3-4	3-4	2-3	3-4
1800	6-7	10-11	3-4	3-4	2-3	4-5
2000	6-7	11-12	4-5	4-5	2-3	4-5
2200	7-8	12-13	4-5	4-5	2-3	6-7
2400	8-9	13-14	4-5	4-5	2-3	7-8
2600	9-10	14-15	5	5	2-3	7-8
2800	9-10	15-16	5	5	2-3	9

You may always choose the high range of vegetables and fruits. Limit your high range selections to only one of the following: meat, bread, milk or fat.

Weekly Progress

_____ Loss _____ Gain _____ Maintain

_____ Attendance _____ Bible Study
_____ Prayer _____ Scripture Reading
_____ Memory Verse _____ CR
_____ Encouragement:
_____ Exercise
_____ Aerobic

_____ Strength _____
_____ Flexibility _____

DAY 5: Date _____

Morning _____

Midday _____

Evening _____

Snacks _____

_____ Meat   ☐ Prayer
_____ Bread   ☐ Bible Study
_____ Vegetable ☐ Scripture Reading
_____ Fruit   ☐ Memory Verse
_____ Milk   ☐ Encouragement
_____ Fat   ☐ Water

Exercise
Aerobic _____

Strength _____
Flexibility _____

DAY 6: Date _____

Morning _____

Midday _____

Evening _____

Snacks _____

_____ Meat   ☐ Prayer
_____ Bread   ☐ Bible Study
_____ Vegetable ☐ Scripture Reading
_____ Fruit   ☐ Memory Verse
_____ Milk   ☐ Encouragement
_____ Fat   ☐ Water

Exercise
Aerobic _____

Strength _____
Flexibility _____

DAY 7: Date _____

Morning _____

Midday _____

Evening _____

Snacks _____

_____ Meat   ☐ Prayer
_____ Bread   ☐ Bible Study
_____ Vegetable ☐ Scripture Reading
_____ Fruit   ☐ Memory Verse
_____ Milk   ☐ Encouragement
_____ Fat   ☐ Water

Exercise
Aerobic _____

Strength _____
Flexibility _____

DAY 1: Date _____

Morning _____

Midday _____

Evening _____

Snacks _____

____ Meat   ☐ Prayer
____ Bread   ☐ Bible Study
____ Vegetable   ☐ Scripture Reading
____ Fruit   ☐ Memory Verse
____ Milk   ☐ Encouragement
____ Fat   ____ Water

Exercise
Aerobic _____
Strength _____
Flexibility _____

DAY 2: Date _____

Morning _____

Midday _____

Evening _____

Snacks _____

____ Meat   ☐ Prayer
____ Bread   ☐ Bible Study
____ Vegetable   ☐ Scripture Reading
____ Fruit   ☐ Memory Verse
____ Milk   ☐ Encouragement
____ Fat   ____ Water

Exercise
Aerobic _____
Strength _____
Flexibility _____

DAY 3: Date _____

Morning _____

Midday _____

Evening _____

Snacks _____

____ Meat   ☐ Prayer
____ Bread   ☐ Bible Study
____ Vegetable   ☐ Scripture Reading
____ Fruit   ☐ Memory Verse
____ Milk   ☐ Encouragement
____ Fat   ____ Water

Exercise
Aerobic _____
Strength _____
Flexibility _____

DAY 4: Date _____

Morning _____

Midday _____

Evening _____

Snacks _____

____ Meat   ☐ Prayer
____ Bread   ☐ Bible Study
____ Vegetable   ☐ Scripture Reading
____ Fruit   ☐ Memory Verse
____ Milk   ☐ Encouragement
____ Fat   ____ Water

Exercise
Aerobic _____
Strength _____
Flexibility _____

FIRST PLACE CR

Name _____

Date _____ through _____

Week # _____ Calorie Level _____

Daily Exchange Plan

Level	Meat	Bread	Veggie	Fruit	Milk	Fat
1200	4-5	5-6	3	2-3	2-3	3-4
1400	5-6	6-7	3-4	3-4	2-3	3-4
1500	5-6	7-8	3-4	3-4	2-3	3-4
1600	6-7	8-9	3-4	3-4	2-3	3-4
1800	6-7	10-11	3-4	3-4	2-3	4-5
2000	6-7	11-12	4-5	4-5	2-3	4-5
2200	7-8	12-13	4-5	4-5	2-3	6-7
2400	8-9	13-14	4-5	4-5	2-3	7-8
2600	9-10	14-15	5	5	2-3	7-8
2800	9-10	15-16	5	5	2-3	9

You may always choose the high range of vegetables and fruits. Limit your high range selections to only one of the following: meat, bread, milk or fat.

Weekly Progress

Loss _____ Gain _____ Maintain _____

____ Attendance   ____ Bible Study
____ Prayer   ____ Scripture Reading
____ Memory Verse ____ CR
____ Encouragement:
____ Exercise
Aerobic _____

Strength _____
Flexibility _____

DAY 5: Date _____

Morning _____

Midday _____

Evening _____

Snacks _____

____ Meat   ☐ Prayer
____ Bread   ☐ Bible Study
____ Vegetable   ☐ Scripture Reading
____ Fruit   ☐ Memory Verse
____ Milk   ☐ Encouragement
____ Fat   ☐ Water

Exercise _____
Aerobic _____

Strength _____
Flexibility _____

DAY 6 Date _____

Morning _____

Midday _____

Evening _____

Snacks _____

____ Meat   ☐ Prayer
____ Bread   ☐ Bible Study
____ Vegetable   ☐ Scripture Reading
____ Fruit   ☐ Memory Verse
____ Milk   ☐ Encouragement
____ Fat   ☐ Water

Exercise _____
Aerobic _____

Strength _____
Flexibility _____

DAY 7: Date _____

Morning _____

Midday _____

Evening _____

Snacks _____

____ Meat   ☐ Prayer
____ Bread   ☐ Bible Study
____ Vegetable   ☐ Scripture Reading
____ Fruit   ☐ Memory Verse
____ Milk   ☐ Encouragement
____ Fat   ☐ Water

Exercise _____
Aerobic _____

Strength _____
Flexibility _____

DAY 1: Date _____

Morning _____

Midday _____

Evening _____

Snacks _____

Meat ____	☐ Prayer
Bread ____	☐ Bible Study
Vegetable ____	☐ Scripture Reading
Fruit ____	☐ Memory Verse
Milk ____	☐ Encouragement
Fat ____	
Water ____	

Exercise
Aerobic _____
Strength _____
Flexibility _____

DAY 2: Date _____

Morning _____

Midday _____

Evening _____

Snacks _____

Meat ____	☐ Prayer
Bread ____	☐ Bible Study
Vegetable ____	☐ Scripture Reading
Fruit ____	☐ Memory Verse
Milk ____	☐ Encouragement
Fat ____	
Water ____	

Exercise
Aerobic _____
Strength _____
Flexibility _____

DAY 3: Date _____

Morning _____

Midday _____

Evening _____

Snacks _____

Meat ____	☐ Prayer
Bread ____	☐ Bible Study
Vegetable ____	☐ Scripture Reading
Fruit ____	☐ Memory Verse
Milk ____	☐ Encouragement
Fat ____	
Water ____	

Exercise
Aerobic _____
Strength _____
Flexibility _____

DAY 4: Date _____

Morning _____

Midday _____

Evening _____

Snacks _____

Meat ____	☐ Prayer
Bread ____	☐ Bible Study
Vegetable ____	☐ Scripture Reading
Fruit ____	☐ Memory Verse
Milk ____	☐ Encouragement
Fat ____	
Water ____	

Exercise
Aerobic _____
Strength _____
Flexibility _____

FIRST PLACE CR

Name _____
Date _____ through _____
Week # _____ Calorie Level _____

Daily Exchange Plan

Level	Meat	Bread	Veggie	Fruit	Milk	Fat
1200	4-5	5-6	3	2-3	2-3	3-4
1400	5-6	6-7	3-4	3-4	2-3	3-4
1500	5-6	7-8	3-4	3-4	2-3	3-4
1600	6-7	8-9	3-4	3-4	2-3	3-4
1800	6-7	10-11	3-4	3-4	2-3	4-5
2000	6-7	11-12	4-5	4-5	2-3	4-5
2200	7-8	12-13	4-5	4-5	2-3	6-7
2400	8-9	13-14	4-5	4-5	2-3	7-8
2600	9-10	14-15	5	5	2-3	7-8
2800	9-10	15-16	5	5	2-3	9

You may always choose the high range of vegetables and fruits. Limit your high range selections to only one of the following: meat, bread, milk or fat.

Weekly Progress

_____ Loss _____ Gain _____ Maintain

_____ Attendance _____ Bible Study
_____ Prayer _____ Scripture Reading
_____ Memory Verse _____ CR
_____ Encouragement:
_____ Exercise
Aerobic _____
Strength _____
Flexibility _____

DAY 7: Date _____

Morning _____

Midday _____

Evening _____

Snacks _____

_____ Meat   ☐ Prayer
_____ Bread   ☐ Bible Study
_____ Vegetable   ☐ Scripture Reading
_____ Fruit   ☐ Memory Verse
_____ Milk   ☐ Encouragement
_____ Fat   ☐ Water
Exercise
Aerobic _____

Strength _____
Flexibility _____

DAY 6: Date _____

Morning _____

Midday _____

Evening _____

Snacks _____

_____ Meat   ☐ Prayer
_____ Bread   ☐ Bible Study
_____ Vegetable   ☐ Scripture Reading
_____ Fruit   ☐ Memory Verse
_____ Milk   ☐ Encouragement
_____ Fat   ☐ Water
Exercise
Aerobic _____

Strength _____
Flexibility _____

DAY 5: Date _____

Morning _____

Midday _____

Evening _____

Snacks _____

_____ Meat   ☐ Prayer
_____ Bread   ☐ Bible Study
_____ Vegetable   ☐ Scripture Reading
_____ Fruit   ☐ Memory Verse
_____ Milk   ☐ Encouragement
_____ Fat   ☐ Water
Exercise
Aerobic _____

Strength _____
Flexibility _____

DAY 1: Date _____

Morning _____

Midday _____

Evening _____

Snacks _____

___ Meat ___	☐ Prayer
___ Bread ___	☐ Bible Study
___ Vegetable ___	☐ Scripture Reading
___ Fruit ___	☐ Memory Verse
___ Milk ___	☐ Encouragement
___ Fat ___ Water ___	

Exercise
Aerobic _____

Strength _____
Flexibility _____

DAY 2: Date _____

Morning _____

Midday _____

Evening _____

Snacks _____

___ Meat ___	☐ Prayer
___ Bread ___	☐ Bible Study
___ Vegetable ___	☐ Scripture Reading
___ Fruit ___	☐ Memory Verse
___ Milk ___	☐ Encouragement
___ Fat ___ Water ___	

Exercise
Aerobic _____

Strength _____
Flexibility _____

DAY 3: Date _____

Morning _____

Midday _____

Evening _____

Snacks _____

___ Meat ___	☐ Prayer
___ Bread ___	☐ Bible Study
___ Vegetable ___	☐ Scripture Reading
___ Fruit ___	☐ Memory Verse
___ Milk ___	☐ Encouragement
___ Fat ___ Water ___	

Exercise
Aerobic _____

Strength _____
Flexibility _____

DAY 4: Date _____

Morning _____

Midday _____

Evening _____

Snacks _____

___ Meat ___	☐ Prayer
___ Bread ___	☐ Bible Study
___ Vegetable ___	☐ Scripture Reading
___ Fruit ___	☐ Memory Verse
___ Milk ___	☐ Encouragement
___ Fat ___ Water ___	

Exercise
Aerobic _____

Strength _____
Flexibility _____

FIRST PLACE CR

Name _____

Daily Exchange Plan

Level	Meat	Bread	Veggie	Fruit	Milk	Fat
1200	4-5	5-6	3	2-3	2-3	3-4
1400	5-6	6-7	3-4	3-4	2-3	3-4
1500	5-6	7-8	3-4	3-4	2-3	3-4
1600	6-7	8-9	3-4	3-4	2-3	3-4
1800	6-7	10-11	3-4	3-4	2-3	4-5
2000	6-7	11-12	4-5	4-5	2-3	4-5
2200	7-8	12-13	4-5	4-5	2-3	6-7
2400	8-9	13-14	4-5	4-5	2-3	7-8
2600	9-10	14-15	5	5	2-3	7-8
2800	9-10	15-16	5	5	2-3	9

You may always choose the high range of vegetables and fruits. Limit your high range selections to only one of the following: meat, bread, milk or fat.

Weekly Progress

_____ Loss _____ Gain _____ Maintain

_____ Attendance _____ Bible Study
_____ Prayer _____ Scripture Reading
_____ Memory Verse _____ CR
_____ Encouragement:
_____ Exercise
_____ Aerobic

Strength _____
Flexibility _____

DAY 5: Date _____

Morning _____
_____

Midday _____
_____

Evening _____
_____

Snacks _____
_____

_____ Meat   ☐ Prayer
_____ Bread   ☐ Bible Study
_____ Vegetable   ☐ Scripture Reading
_____ Fruit   ☐ Memory Verse
_____ Milk   ☐ Encouragement
_____ Fat   Water _____

Exercise
Aerobic _____

Strength _____
Flexibility _____

DAY 6: Date _____

Morning _____
_____

Midday _____
_____

Evening _____
_____

Snacks _____
_____

_____ Meat   ☐ Prayer
_____ Bread   ☐ Bible Study
_____ Vegetable   ☐ Scripture Reading
_____ Fruit   ☐ Memory Verse
_____ Milk   ☐ Encouragement:
_____ Fat   Water _____

Exercise
Aerobic _____

Strength _____
Flexibility _____

DAY 7: Date _____

Morning _____
_____

Midday _____
_____

Evening _____
_____

Snacks _____
_____

_____ Meat   ☐ Prayer
_____ Bread   ☐ Bible Study
_____ Vegetable   ☐ Scripture Reading
_____ Fruit   ☐ Memory Verse
_____ Milk   ☐ Encouragement
_____ Fat   Water _____

Exercise
Aerobic _____

Strength _____
Flexibility _____

DAY 1: Date _____

Morning _____

Midday _____

Evening _____

Snacks _____

____ Meat	☐ Prayer
____ Bread	☐ Bible Study
____ Vegetable	☐ Scripture Reading
____ Fruit	☐ Memory Verse
____ Milk	☐ Encouragement
____ Fat ____ Water	

Exercise
Aerobic _____

Strength _____
Flexibility _____

DAY 2: Date _____

Morning _____

Midday _____

Evening _____

Snacks _____

____ Meat	☐ Prayer
____ Bread	☐ Bible Study
____ Vegetable	☐ Scripture Reading
____ Fruit	☐ Memory Verse
____ Milk	☐ Encouragement
____ Fat ____ Water	

Exercise
Aerobic _____

Strength _____
Flexibility _____

DAY 3: Date _____

Morning _____

Midday _____

Evening _____

Snacks _____

____ Meat	☐ Prayer
____ Bread	☐ Bible Study
____ Vegetable	☐ Scripture Reading
____ Fruit	☐ Memory Verse
____ Milk	☐ Encouragement
____ Fat ____ Water	

Exercise
Aerobic _____

Strength _____
Flexibility _____

DAY 4: Date _____

Morning _____

Midday _____

Evening _____

Snacks _____

____ Meat	☐ Prayer
____ Bread	☐ Bible Study
____ Vegetable	☐ Scripture Reading
____ Fruit	☐ Memory Verse
____ Milk	☐ Encouragement
____ Fat ____ Water	

Exercise
Aerobic _____

Strength _____
Flexibility _____

Name _____

Date _____ through _____

Week # _____ Calorie Level _____

Daily Exchange Plan

Level	Meat	Bread	Veggie	Fruit	Milk	Fat
1200	4-5	5-6	3	2-3	2-3	3-4
1400	5-6	6-7	3-4	3-4	2-3	3-4
1500	5-6	7-8	3-4	3-4	2-3	3-4
1600	6-7	8-9	3-4	3-4	2-3	3-4
1800	6-7	10-11	3-4	3-4	2-3	4-5
2000	6-7	11-12	4-5	4-5	2-3	4-5
2200	7-8	12-13	4-5	4-5	2-3	6-7
2400	8-9	13-14	4-5	4-5	2-3	7-8
2600	9-10	14-15	5	5	2-3	7-8
2800	9-10	15-16	5	5	2-3	9

You may always choose the high range of vegetables and fruits. Limit your high range selections to only one of the following: meat, bread, milk or fat.

Weekly Progress

_____ Loss _____ Gain _____ Maintain

_____ Attendance _____ Bible Study
_____ Prayer _____ Scripture Reading
_____ Memory Verse _____ CR
_____ Encouragement:
_____ Exercise
Aerobic _____

_____ Strength _____
_____ Flexibility _____

DAY 7: Date _____

Morning _____

Midday _____

Evening _____

Snacks _____

_____ Meat   ☐ Prayer
_____ Bread   ☐ Bible Study
_____ Vegetable ☐ Scripture Reading
_____ Fruit   ☐ Memory Verse
_____ Milk   ☐ Encouragement
_____ Fat   _____ Water

Exercise
Aerobic _____

Strength _____
Flexibility _____

DAY 6: Date _____

Morning _____

Midday _____

Evening _____

Snacks _____

_____ Meat   ☐ Prayer
_____ Bread   ☐ Bible Study
_____ Vegetable ☐ Scripture Reading
_____ Fruit   ☐ Memory Verse
_____ Milk   ☐ Encouragement
_____ Fat   _____ Water

Exercise
Aerobic _____

Strength _____
Flexibility _____

DAY 5: Date _____

Morning _____

Midday _____

Evening _____

Snacks _____

_____ Meat   ☐ Prayer
_____ Bread   ☐ Bible Study
_____ Vegetable ☐ Scripture Reading
_____ Fruit   ☐ Memory Verse
_____ Milk   ☐ Encouragement
_____ Fat   _____ Water

Exercise
Aerobic _____

Strength _____
Flexibility _____

DAY 1: Date _____

Morning _____

Midday _____

Evening _____

Snacks _____

____ Meat	☐ Prayer
____ Bread	☐ Bible Study
____ Vegetable	☐ Scripture Reading
____ Fruit	☐ Memory Verse
____ Milk	☐ Encouragement
____ Fat	____ Water

Exercise

Aerobic _____

Strength _____

Flexibility _____

DAY 2: Date _____

Morning _____

Midday _____

Evening _____

Snacks _____

____ Meat	☐ Prayer
____ Bread	☐ Bible Study
____ Vegetable	☐ Scripture Reading
____ Fruit	☐ Memory Verse
____ Milk	☐ Encouragement
____ Fat	____ Water

Exercise

Aerobic _____

Strength _____

Flexibility _____

DAY 3: Date _____

Morning _____

Midday _____

Evening _____

Snacks _____

____ Meat	☐ Prayer
____ Bread	☐ Bible Study
____ Vegetable	☐ Scripture Reading
____ Fruit	☐ Memory Verse
____ Milk	☐ Encouragement
____ Fat	____ Water

Exercise

Aerobic _____

Strength _____

Flexibility _____

DAY 4: Date _____

Morning _____

Midday _____

Evening _____

Snacks _____

____ Meat	☐ Prayer
____ Bread	☐ Bible Study
____ Vegetable	☐ Scripture Reading
____ Fruit	☐ Memory Verse
____ Milk	☐ Encouragement
____ Fat	____ Water

Exercise

Aerobic _____

Strength _____

Flexibility _____

FIRST PLACE CR

Name _____

Date _____ through _____

Week # _____ Calorie Level _____

Daily Exchange Plan

Level	Meat	Bread	Veggie	Fruit	Milk	Fat
1200	4-5	5-6	3	2-3	2-3	3-4
1400	5-6	6-7	3-4	3-4	2-3	3-4
1500	5-6	7-8	3-4	3-4	2-3	3-4
1600	6-7	8-9	3-4	3-4	2-3	3-4
1800	6-7	10-11	3-4	3-4	2-3	4-5
2000	6-7	11-12	4-5	4-5	2-3	4-5
2200	7-8	12-13	4-5	4-5	2-3	6-7
2400	8-9	13-14	4-5	4-5	2-3	7-8
2600	9-10	14-15	5	5	2-3	7-8
2800	9-10	15-16	5	5	2-3	9

You may always choose the high range of vegetables and fruits. Limit your high range selections to only one of the following: meat, bread, milk or fat.

Weekly Progress

_____ Loss _____ Gain _____ Maintain

_____ Attendance _____ Bible Study
_____ Prayer _____ Scripture Reading
_____ Memory Verse _____ CR
_____ Encouragement:
_____ Exercise
Aerobic _____
_____
Strength _____
Flexibility _____

DAY 5: Date _____

Morning _____
_____

Midday _____
_____

Evening _____
_____

Snacks _____
_____

_____ Meat   ☐ Prayer
_____ Bread ☐ Bible Study
_____ Vegetable ☐ Scripture Reading
_____ Fruit ☐ Memory Verse
_____ Milk ☐ Encouragement
_____ Fat _____ Water

Exercise
Aerobic _____

Strength _____
Flexibility _____

DAY 6: Date _____

Morning _____
_____

Midday _____
_____

Evening _____
_____

Snacks _____
_____

_____ Meat   ☐ Prayer
_____ Bread ☐ Bible Study
_____ Vegetable ☐ Scripture Reading
_____ Fruit ☐ Memory Verse
_____ Milk ☐ Encouragement
_____ Fat _____ Water

Exercise
Aerobic _____

Strength _____
Flexibility _____

DAY 7: Date _____

Morning _____
_____

Midday _____
_____

Evening _____
_____

Snacks _____
_____

_____ Meat   ☐ Prayer
_____ Bread ☐ Bible Study
_____ Vegetable ☐ Scripture Reading
_____ Fruit ☐ Memory Verse
_____ Milk ☐ Encouragement
_____ Fat _____ Water

Exercise
Aerobic _____

Strength _____
Flexibility _____

DAY 1: Date _____

Morning _____

Midday _____

Evening _____

Snacks _____

___ Meat	☐ Prayer
___ Bread	☐ Bible Study
___ Vegetable	☐ Scripture Reading
___ Fruit	☐ Memory Verse
___ Milk	☐ Encouragement
___ Fat	___ Water

Exercise
Aerobic _____
Strength _____
Flexibility _____

DAY 2: Date _____

Morning _____

Midday _____

Evening _____

Snacks _____

___ Meat	☐ Prayer
___ Bread	☐ Bible Study
___ Vegetable	☐ Scripture Reading
___ Fruit	☐ Memory Verse
___ Milk	☐ Encouragement
___ Fat	___ Water

Exercise
Aerobic _____
Strength _____
Flexibility _____

DAY 3: Date _____

Morning _____

Midday _____

Evening _____

Snacks _____

___ Meat	☐ Prayer
___ Bread	☐ Bible Study
___ Vegetable	☐ Scripture Reading
___ Fruit	☐ Memory Verse
___ Milk	☐ Encouragement
___ Fat	___ Water

Exercise
Aerobic _____
Strength _____
Flexibility _____

DAY 4: Date _____

Morning _____

Midday _____

Evening _____

Snacks _____

___ Meat	☐ Prayer
___ Bread	☐ Bible Study
___ Vegetable	☐ Scripture Reading
___ Fruit	☐ Memory Verse
___ Milk	☐ Encouragement
___ Fat	___ Water

Exercise
Aerobic _____
Strength _____
Flexibility _____

CONTRIBUTORS

Elizabeth Crews, the writer of the Wellness Worksheets for this study, has a master's degree in Counseling/Psychology/Family Systems Theory, and is a licensed Drug and Alcohol counselor and educator. For 15 years Elizabeth taught small groups and adult Sunday school classes, while also serving as an elder for adult education in her local church. Currently, she leads a First Place group and is a networking leader.

Scott Wilson, C.P.C., C.E.C., A.A.C., the author of the menu plans for this study, is the national food consultant for First Place. Scott is a certified personal chef with the United States Personal Chef Association (USPCA) and is currently serving in the USPCA as chair of the National Advisory Council. He is also a certified executive chef, member of the American Academy of Chefs (AAC) and a member of the American Culinary Federation (ACF). In addition to his role as a personal chef, Scott also serves as an instructor for the Culinary Business Academy of Atlanta, is on the Culinary Advisory Board of the Art Institute of Atlanta and has recently become the Southeast demonstrator chef for AGA Ranges USA. Scott has published three cookbooks and lives in Cumming, Georgia, with his wife, Jennifer, and their daughter, Katie.

Memory Verses

Week One

Then you will know the truth, and the truth will set you free (John 8:32).

Week Two

Surely the arm of the Lord is not too short to save, nor his ear too dull to hear (Isaiah 59:1).

Week Three

Like a city whose walls are broken down is a man who lacks self-control (Proverbs 25:28).

Week Four

But you are a shield around me, O Lord; you bestow glory on me and lift up my head (Psalm 3:3).

Week Five

Humble yourselves, therefore, under God's mighty hand, that he may lift you up in due time (1 Peter 5:6).

Week Six

Devote yourselves to prayer, being watchful and thankful (Colossians 4:2).

Week Seven

You were running a good race. Who cut in on you and kept you from obeying the truth (Galatians 5:7)?

Week Eight

Never be lacking in zeal, but keep your spiritual fervor, serving the Lord (Romans 12:11).

Week Nine

Above all else, guard your heart, for it is the wellspring of life (Proverbs 4:23).

Week Ten

Then a cloud appeared and enveloped them, and a voice came from the cloud: "This is my Son, whom I love. Listen to him" (Mark 9:7)!

THE BIBLE-BASED WEIGHT-LOSS PROGRAM USED SUCCESSFULLY BY OVER A HALF MILLION PEOPLE!

Are you one of the millions of disheartened dieters who've tried one fad diet after another without success? If so, your search for a successful diet is over! But First Place does much more than help you take off weight and keep it off. This Bible-based program will transform your life in every way—physically, mentally, spiritually and emotionally. Now's the time to join!

ESSENTIAL FIRST PLACE PROGRAM MATERIALS

Group Leaders Need:

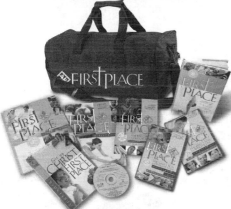

■ **Group Starter Kit** • *ISBN 08307.33698*

This kit has everything group leaders need to help others change their lives forever by giving Christ first place!

Kit includes:

- *Leader's Guide*
- *Member's Guide*
- *First Place* by Carole Lewis with Terry Whalin
- *Giving Christ First Place* Bible Study with Scripture Memory Music CD
- *Introduction to First Place and Nine Commitments* DVD
- *Orientation and Food Exchange Plan* DVD
- *Leadership Training* DVD
- myfirstplace.org three-month trial subscription
- One package of 25 *First Place Brochures*

Group Members Need:

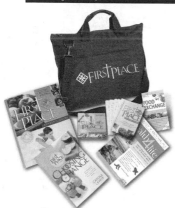

■ **Member's Kit** • *ISBN 08307.33701*

All the material is easy to understand and spells out principles members can easily apply in their daily lives.

Kit includes:

- *Member's Guide* • *Choosing to Change* by Carole Lewis
- *Motivational CDs* • *Food Exchange Pocket Guide*
- *Commitment Records* • *Health 4 Life*
- Scripture Memory Verses

Available where Christian books are sold or by calling 1-800-4-GOSPEL. **Join the First Place community and order products at www.firstplace.org.**

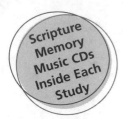
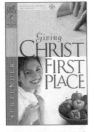
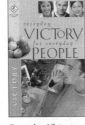
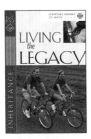
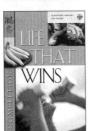
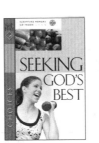
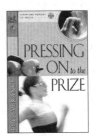
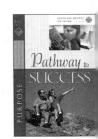
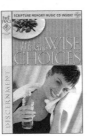
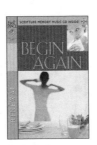
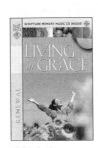
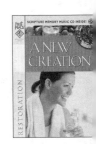
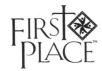